WELCOME TO
BISCUIT LAND

WELCOME TO BISCUIT LAND

A Year in the Life of Touretteshero

JESSICA THOM

Souvenir Press

For Leftwing Idiot who helped me find my power.

In 2010 Jessica Thom set up Touretteshero, an organisation that celebrates the humour and creativity of Tourettes without mocking or self-pity – it's about reclaiming the most frequently misunderstood syndrome on the planet and changing the world one tic at a time.

ACKNOWLEDGEMENTS

Touretteshero exists as an organisation because of the vision, dedication and persuasiveness of my co-founder Matthew Pountney.

Matthew helped me see the creative value of Tourettes where previously I'd seen only problems. Touretteshero and this book would never have happened without him, and my life would have been infinitely tougher. I searched through over 11,000 emails from him and found the one where he first suggests working together to celebrate my tics. It ends: 'It would genuinely be amazing. We could really make something brilliant and funny. Think about it.'

I did, and together we've created something of which I'm very proud.

In addition to Matthew, Michael Pountney and Liz Fraser have helped edit this book from the outset. Their hard work and skill have shaped it. Their encouragement and commitment have enabled me to share my experiences and thoughts during both difficult and exciting times.

Thanks to Souvenir Press for publishing this book and for guiding us through the process. To UnLtd for giving the grant that allowed us to develop the website. To Claire Ball and her colleagues at Tourettes Action. To Daytrippers for supporting the idea – and us.

Touretteshero has been a collaborative project from the outset, and huge numbers of people have helped us build an organisation out of an idea. Particular thanks to: Annie Pender for my stunning superhero suit, Rikki Marr for our logo, Dan Farrow and Matthew Avery for persevering and creating our website. To

Gabriel 'Heatwave' Myddelton for my first Twitter tutorial. To Sam Robinson, Ginny Pickles, Olive Johnson, Keir Williams and Adam Charvet for always answering the phone and doing us a million favours.

To Cassetteboy, The 2 Bears, Al Tourettes and Mr Hay, thanks for turning tics into tunes. And to the NHS and my local social services team, thanks for stopping tics becoming lasting injuries.

Thanks also to my boss, colleagues and all the children at Oasis Children's Venture for making my day job such a joy and supporting me in my 'secret' role as a superhero.

I'm very grateful to Stephen Fry for writing the foreword to this book and giving me (and my tics) an opportunity to contribute to his programme on language.

Huge thanks to all those who feature in the book and who make my life in Biscuit Land such a happy one: to Fat Sister, King Russell, Poppy, Ruth, Laura, Ruby, Emma, Owain, Kyle, Hannah, Fran, Bunny, Harry, the two Ollies, Mum, Dad and Thump-A-Youth Man.

To all the strangers who've offered spontaneous support, insight or kindness, thank you. To those who've done the opposite, you too have contributed to Touretteshero by making it necessary for me to develop the confidence, understanding and humour to challenge you to see things differently.

Thank you to everyone who's helping us 'change the world one tic at a time'.

CONTENTS

FOREWORD

I'm so happy that Jess 'Biscuit' Thom has asked me to write a few words of introduction to this delightful book.

For a quarter of a century Tourettes Syndrome, a neurological dysfunction that presents in the form of involuntary tics, movements and unfiltered utterances, has been a staple of the kind of 'freak show TV' of which producers should be most ashamed. Not more than 10% of Touretters evince 'coprolalia', the propensity willy nilly to blurt out offensive, blasphemous and obscene language, but it is that facet of the syndrome that has almost always taken up the world's attention.

There are those who, for understandable reasons, are deeply offended by this trashy voyeuristic attitude and who point out both how much more common a disorder Tourettes is than was previously thought and how small the minority is who exhibit the telegenic and often hilarious (it must be admitted, even if shamefully) symptom of crude linguistic outbursts. Perhaps nearly as many as 5% of children worldwide suffer from the chronic motor and vocal tics that characterise the condition, and yet for most of us it is only the potty-mouthed 10% of these who interest us and who therefore wrongly define and symbolise the whole syndrome.

When I set out with JP Davidson and Helen Williamson to make *Planet Word*, a series of programmes for the BBC about language, one of the aspects we were very keen to explore was the arena of the forbidden. In short, swearing. Since we are all inside society it is very hard to be objective about the deep-rooted taboos and fears that all of us share. The use of the F, C and more recently N words in our culture still causes many to blench. Why is it that some people, when laid low by strokes that cause almost total language loss or 'aphasia', are able only to blurt out (much to their own discomfort in many cases) the words least tolerable to society's ears? Why do women in childbirth so commonly scream out the most extreme profanities? And why should it be that a neurological disorder like Tourettes Syndrome should cause this, albeit small, minority to pepper their language with involuntary swear words and embarrassingly inappropriate obscenities?

It was quite a journey researching this. It turns out that swearing has a demonstrably analgesic effect, which explains why we curse when we hit our thumbs with a hammer and why those respectable women yell out such shocking curses in childbirth. Even more interestingly, it seems that each culture privileges certain words with extra power: children unswervingly and unnervingly pick up on these so quickly from their parents and peers that very early on in the language acquisition process these special words (usually to do with pee, poo and procreation) are 'stored' in a special place, a region of the brain deeper within the primal emotional wiring of the basal ganglia, and not in the 'higher cognitive' areas where everyday words are thought to be transcribed. And this seems to be why they come out under stress and pressure or as a result of special dysfunctions such as Tourettes, which side-step the brain's usual monitoring system. In other words, Tourettes, acute pain and damage from certain localised cerebral haemorrhages or infarctions seem to bypass the usual censoring mechanisms that inhibit our access to the obscene words buried deep within us.

Of course plenty of us swear all the time amongst our peers, but only the rudest or most eccentric (yes, Brian Blessed, I am looking at you) are unable to moderate their language when in the presence of those whom we might guess will be offended. We may wear jeans and hoodies on informal occasions and yet be perfectly capable of wearing a suit or even dinner jacket or ball gown should the occasion demand. In other words, most of us can consciously select our verbal dress too, our discourse and how slangy or sweary it is. The few with Tourettes-related copro-lalia don't have that choice, and while it may be amusing (and has, it must be acknowledged, given rise to a very funny t-shirt – a quick google of 'Tourettes t-shirt' will reveal it) and remains an endless source of popular television, for those who live with it every day, either as friends and family or as one actually with the condition, there comes a time when the laughter stops.

I was rather dreading a conversation with a Touretter and/or their parent. Some people who had heard that the subject of swearing was going to be included in my programme had already got in touch with me via Twitter and the usual channels to give me a good telling off before we had even started. If I was told once that Tourettes was not about swearing and that if dared go down the usual path I should lose all credibility, I was told a hundred times.

'How are we going to manage this,' we asked ourselves, 'with-out looking over-earnest and politically correct on the one hand or crassly vulgar and scientifically simplistic on the other?'

Enter the blessed Jess Thom. We heard about Jess and her Touretteshero project through Twitter. Plenty of her admirers eventually got through to me, showing me links to her website, and she was happy to take part in the programme and explain her experience and her unique and inspiring way of dealing with it.

Here was someone, unquestionably a member of that ten per-cent group, who chose to embrace the condition, to be open, funny, frank, intelligent and enchantingly entertaining about it. With dash, panache, chic, élan and lots of other qualities that sound like makes of perfume, Jess transforms herself into a superhero in order to educate children and others who know nothing about the condition and to empower those who do have it and to encourage them not to feel ashamed, guilty or cursed.

Tourettes, by virtue of its lack of inhibition and filtering, gives rise to extraordinary collisions of image and category. These are wonderful springboards to art and surreal humour. Jess encourages fellow Touretters to write down their phrases and outbursts and translate the imagery into surprising and intriguing sculptures, collages and pictures. A kind of aleatory art which doesn't need opiates or hallucinogens to kickstart it.

Jess's merry cry of 'Biscuit, biscuit, biscuit!' delighted, amused and touched all who watched *Planet Word*. The sight of her pounding her own chest as she spoke caused many of us to wince in sympathy too, for surely the battering she gives herself every day must cause bruising and pain. But Jess is not the kind to invite sympathy: self-pity is not part of her make-up. She recognises, as do her family, the differences between Tourettes-inspired swearing and the more 'voluntary' swearing she might, like anyone her age, sometimes be guilty of. Her wit, her sparkle and her courage enlivened what could otherwise have been a delicate, turgid or prurient section of our film. For that we are all grateful.

Now she has been and gone and done and written this charming, touching and valuable book. I hope reading it will give you an insight into the life of someone who might, statistically speaking, have expected her Tourettes to fall back as she grew into adulthood as it often typically can, but has had to cope with the fact that in her case the condition seems to hold her as fast as ever it did. She cheerfully accepts her lot, and as a way of coping herself and a way of helping others to cope has been brave enough to share her world. She also allows us to smile and laugh without feeling guilty of mocking and that is a supremely graceful gift from her to the world.

Jess is a true hero, with or without her Touretteshero costume. Jess fuck biscuit Thom, I biscuit fuck fuck biscuit salute biscuit you.

Stephen Fry

JANUARY

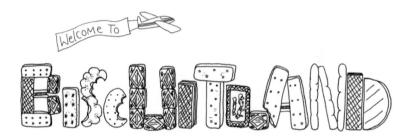

24 HOURS OF NOISE

It's the start of a new year and I've decided it's time to recognise and record something that's a big part of my life, but that I've always tried to ignore.

So I've bought a voice recorder, and for the next 24 hours I'm going to record every noise I make.

You might think this'll be pretty boring since I'll be on my own all day, but I know it won't because I've got Tourettes Syndrome. This means I make involuntary noises and movements, and say things I can't control – all the time. Although I don't know exactly what I'll be saying, I know it'll be a lot, and some of it'll be very funny.

From this point on Tourettes won't be my problem – it'll be my power. From now on, I'm going to be Touretteshero.

WELCOME TO BISCUIT LAND

This is a place for me to share and celebrate the creativity and humour of Tourettes with you. It's not about mocking or commiserating. It's about reclaiming the most frequently mis-understood syndrome on the planet.

Tourettes is a mysterious neurological condition. Having it means I make movements and noises I can't control – these are called tics. Sometimes they're simple and just involve me squeaking or nodding my head. Sometimes, though, they're more complicated and involve me saying stuff like 'Sexually frustrated dog food'. And that's when it gets interesting.

No one really knows what causes Tourettes, but it's believed to be an inherited genetic condition involving an imbalance in the function of the brain's neurotransmitters. It's thought that between 200,000 and 300,000 people in the UK have Tourettes to one degree or another. When I say people, it's mainly men – about four times more men than women in fact. So that means I really stand out.

All my tics are involuntary and I tic hundreds of times a day, so I'm rarely still or quiet.

'There's a barn dance in my mind.'

Tourettes is pretty much the only special power I'll ever need. Like most special powers, it gives me extraordinary abilities that can be used for good, but it also brings incredible challenges. In this diary I'll be sharing some of the best and worst bits of Tourettes.

'There's a beaver in my bum writing an essay about dogs.'

What follows contains language some people might find offensive. Only 10% of people with Tourettes swear involuntarily, but I'm one of them. So if you're easily offended, this isn't the book for you.

If not, welcome to my mind.

MY HEROES

Despite my superhero status, I'm not really the 'lone vigilante' type. Many of my friends and family will be cropping up throughout the blog. Today I'm going to introduce five of them you should know about from the start.

Leftwing Idiot's a close friend and neighbour whom I've known for 10 *long* years. 'Leftwing Idiot' is something I used to say as a tic that seemed to be triggered by him. Although he's not usually an idiot, he is prone to the occasional leftwing rant. Generally though he's incredibly supportive and understanding of my Tourettes. Occasionally he finds it irritating and frustrating, but most of the time he just finds it funny. A while ago he used to try and programme me to say stuff by repeating it over and over again. Annoyingly, it often worked. He doesn't do that so much any more.

Fat Sister's my actual sister, but she's not actually fat. Leftwing Idiot programmed me to say 'Fat Sister' as a tic when she was on a diet once, and eventually it stuck. Fat Sister's younger than me and doesn't have Tourettes. Nothing fazes Fat Sister – she's always matter-of-fact about my Tourettes and pretty unshakable in general. She works as a hospital doctor for the NHS and we live together, along with her boyfriend King Russell. When we were children Fat Sister used to be on the receiving end of lots of my tics, some of which were quite intrusive, like me biting her arm at breakfast. She barely seemed to notice most of the time, despite how odd and sometimes painful it must have been.

King Russell's been going out with Fat Sister since they were both teenagers. He lives with us in the Touretteshero lair. 'King Russell' is one of many Russell-related tics. He's done everything from breaking the shower to falling out of a wormhole. He fully embraces his tic-name and encourages its use at every opportunity.

Poppy is Leftwing Idiot's girlfriend and she's amazing. She's a relatively recent addition to the Touretteshero team but we've quickly become good friends. She's embraced a life enriched by tics and loves looking through the notebook where I write them all down. In the time we've known each other Poppy's shown me incredible kindness and support.

Apart from people on TV and my own reflection in the mirror, Ruth is the first person with Tourettes I ever encountered. We met about a year ago and I was instantly struck by how similar our tics are. We've been friends ever since and often go on mischievous expeditions together on the understanding that those who tic together stick together.

LONG DIVISION AND THATCHER

For the last five years I've kept track of my regular tics, the ones I say or do over and over again (for months or even years on end). Until now, though, I've never paid much attention to the tics I *don't* repeat all the time. These occur every day, and I might only say them once or a handful of times. Some can be linked to or triggered by specific situations or sounds, but the majority are random. Recently, I've started to record these one-off tics. Below is today's selection:

'Careless whisper costs £1.'
'Long division killed your soul.'
'Joy Division killed your soul.'
'Jim Davidson killed your soul.'
'Les Dennis or Margaret Thatcher? Choose.'

As you can see, it's fairly random stuff. I can state with confidence that I wasn't consciously thinking about any of these things when I said them. Some people describe Tourettes as saying what you're thinking, but for me this doesn't ring true, and it oversimplifies something I've always found complex and mystifying.

This doesn't mean my tics are never triggered by things I've seen, thought or heard, because sometimes they are – but I still wouldn't describe it as saying what I'm thinking. The vast majority of my tics tend not to be triggered by events or my surroundings at all, and a lot of them are completely inoffensive:

'Squirrel.'
'Daisy.'
'Sellotape.'
'Biscuit.'

However, some *are* offensive:

'Pony cunt.'
'Poirot pubes.'
'Fuck a shed.'

Some of my tics can be pretty complex:

'Tony Blair sucks cock through his tiny mouth.'
'Alexa Chung died. She stubbed her toe on the edge of the world.'
'Take a picture of your mum's best friend wintering in Lebanon, naked in a bath.'

Sometimes a tic will come out in two or more parts:

'Squirrels ejaculate – over their mums – on Sundays.'

Or it will be a response to a previous tic:

'Russell broke the shower ...'
'... but he didn't shoot the deputy.'

They also evolve, and go through distinct phases over several months:

'Dog.'
'Dogfood.'
'Dogfish.'
'Fish.'
'Fishing.'

Some phrases are linked to themes, words, or sounds:

'God loves gerbils.'
'God loves sandwiches.'
'God loves everyone – except you.'

What I struggle to get my head around is that while my tics aren't a reflection of what I'm thinking, they clearly draw on things I know, or that I'm aware of, or have thought about at some point in my life. All these unconnected things get jumbled around and spat out again. They're often random but they're rarely incoherent.

I don't usually know I've ticced until immediately after it's come out, but I can sometimes stop myself halfway through. If I catch a tic that isn't a regular before it's complete I've no idea what it would've been if I'd let it continue.

Why certain words become regular tics is a mystery to me. They become fixed features in my life and can usually be linked to certain times or experiences. If I think back I can date the start of my regular tics by using memories of places, people or events. I often notice that I've stopped saying a certain word or making a certain movement when something else has taken its place.

Tics that are phrases are often funny and create interesting imagery. However, by themselves they don't give the full picture of Tourettes, as they're often accompanied by other sounds and movements which vary a lot.

One medical handbook describes Tourettes tics as: 'Irrepressible, explosive, occasionally obscene verbal ejaculations.' It goes on to say: 'There may be a witty, innovatory, phantasmagoric picture, with mimicry, antics, playfulness, extravagance, impudence, audacity, dramatisations, surreal associations, uninhibited effect.' (*Oxford Handbook of Clinical Medicine*, Eighth Edition: Murray Longmore, Ian Wilkinson, Edward Davidson, Alexander Foulkes and Ahmad Mafi, Oxford Handbooks Series.)

I like this definition because it recognises aspects of Tourettes that often get lost in other descriptions.

There are many unanswered questions about Tourettes, and I expect the journey we'll go on will unearth even more. Hopefully, this diary will provide a place to reflect on and enjoy plenty of 'witty, audacious and surreal' tics.

DISCLOSURE

Some people are surprised when they find out I have a job. My tics are very noticeable, so people sometimes assume I'm not able to work or that I'm not employable.

As it turns out, I'm very employable, and after nearly three years with my current employers I'm preparing for a big change and a new job. I'm looking forward to the challenges of a different role and I'm gearing up to introduce a whole fresh bunch of people to all my tics.

I'm starting in about a month. My boss-to-be knows I have Tourettes because I wrote it on my application form and I met her at my interview.

This evening, when I went to deliver some documents to her, I asked her if she was ready for Tourettes. She said confidently, 'Yes, it's not a problem.'

GOD SAYS

Leftwing Idiot's back in London. He's been away for a bit, so to celebrate his return I took round too much Indian food and his Christmas present. Leftwing Idiot's been a good friend for many years and he's given me masses of support. Every now and again he's suggested I do something creative with my tics, but for a long time I'd dismissed this idea out of hand. I didn't see why anyone else would be interested.

But last summer a new set of tics arrived themed around God, and Leftwing Idiot suggested they might make good slogans for the posters you find outside churches. I thought this could work so I created a set of prints called 'God Says'. While Leftwing Idiot was away I finished the series and had one of them printed and mounted for him.

That was the present I gave him this evening to thank him for all his encouragement. It reads:

'God loves you except if you're a cunt.'

CEASEFIRE

I was walking home quite late last night and there were two men fighting on the street. As I approached, squeaking, they both stopped and looked at me. One of them asked very directly, 'What's that about then?' I said, 'Tourettes Syndrome.' He smiled broadly and said, 'Is that what you've got?' I confirmed this and he reached out and slapped me on the back and said, 'Good girl.' We both continued on our way in opposite directions. A few moments later, I heard a bang and turned round to see one of the men rebounding off a bus stop.

NO ANGEL

Ruth texted me earlier to ask if I wanted to join her and some friends for a drink tonight. I was totally up for it, but the only thing putting me off was the journey. Having Tourettes and using public transport can be a gruelling combination. It's hard enough trying to get my hands to hold on to anything long enough to keep me steady without having to worry about the unpredictable reactions of other passengers.

I wasn't sure if I could face travelling across London on my own. But I wanted to see Ruth so I set off by tube for North London to meet her. The journey was going well until one stop before where I'd planned to get off. The driver announced that Angel station was closed due to flooding, so I got off at Old Street and went up the escalator.

I approached two members of staff who were standing together by the ticket barriers and asked one of them for the best way to get to Angel. He ignored me, so I asked again, but he turned his back on me to speak to another passenger. I moved round and explained that I had Tourettes, that if I was swearing or making unusual movements they were not directed at him, and that I just needed some information. He looked at me and said, 'I'm not giving you any fucking information.'

I was shocked and asked him why he'd sworn at me like that. He didn't answer and just walked away. I tried again to explain about Tourettes but he continued to ignore me. I realised that trying to make him understand was pointless and decided it would be best to find someone else to help, but the other member of staff had gone away.

I tried to get through the ticket barrier, but when I swiped my freedom pass it didn't work so I had to go back to the same member of staff and ask him to let me out. He said he would let me through when I stopped swearing. I started to cry and said, 'I can't stop swearing – I've got Tourettes Syndrome.' He walked away again and left me in tears, stuck behind the barrier.

I felt humiliated and didn't know what to do so I called out to anyone in the ticket hall for assistance. I shouted, 'I need help to get out and this man isn't helping me.' Most people walked past and I began to sob. A woman on the other side of the barrier came over and asked what was happening. I couldn't tell her straightaway because I was so upset. The member of staff who'd refused to help me pointed at a side gate and said, 'Tell her to go over there.' I walked round and spoke briefly to the woman who'd helped me.

When I stopped crying I approached the ticket office to make a complaint and get the directions I needed. The man at the desk listened politely and said he'd call the station supervisor. This turned out to be the man who'd gone away when I first asked for directions.

I explained that I had Tourettes and described what had just happened. I asked him to write down the name of the member of staff who'd sworn at me but he refused, saying he didn't have to give that information to me. He went on, 'If you want to make a complaint, you know the station and the time.' I asked if he would write down his own name, but he said, 'You can see it here', pointing to his badge. I asked him again and he reluctantly wrote his first name on the back of an old receipt.

I left the station and found the quietest place I could to call Leftwing Idiot. To start with I described what had happened calmly, but as I repeated what the man had said I broke down again. I didn't feel like going out any more and couldn't face getting back on public transport, so I decided to take a cab home. I called Ruth, and sadly she understood all too well how it felt to be treated in this way.

The cab came and as soon as I got in I began to explain my tics to the driver. Before I'd finished he stopped me and said, 'You've got Tourettes. No worries here – my best mate of twenty years has Tourettes, you're in the right cab.' And I was. He was brilliant, and by the time I got home I felt much calmer and more cheerful. I went to Leftwing Idiot's and hung out with him and some other friends.

I can understand that if you've not met someone with Tourettes before some tics can be challenging. But it's really not right for people working with the public to be disrespectful and unhelpful.

I've already written a letter to Transport for London to complain – it'll be interesting to see how they respond.

SHE'S ONLY GOT TOURETTES

The rain was thumping down as I walked along Brixton High Street tonight and the traffic was moving at a crawl. The pavement was crowded and lots of people were staring nervously at me. A passing cyclist, weaving through the traffic wearing a fluorescent waterproof, shouted out to some anxious pedestrians, 'Don't be scared, she's only got Tourettes.'

SNOW DAY

London is still, or at least very slow, because it's been snowing heavily. I'm not still, but that's normal for me. The snow's given me an unexpected day off so I've decided to listen to and transcribe the recording I made of myself on New Year's Day.

I wasn't surprised by my vocal tics when I played them back, but I hadn't expected to hear the sounds of my motor tics – the mic had picked up all the times I thumped my chest, which was 130 in the first hour.

I've no idea what, if anything, I'm going to do with this recording but I decided to see if I could get a measure of how often I tic because I find it very hard to tell whether they're becoming more frequent or not. Tourettes changes over time and my tics are likely to keep going up and down in intensity and frequency throughout my life.

I've had tics since I was a child. My first memory of not being able to stop squeaking was when I was about six. My tics then were much less obvious than they are now, but I still worried about how I moved and I used to get upset when I behaved in an erratic way because I didn't understand what was happening. By my late teens I knew I probably had Tourettes but I didn't feel able to talk to anyone about it.

When I left home I moved into a shared house with Laura and Emma, who are still two of my closest friends. Emma's room was next to mine and she used to complain about the noise of my bed moving about and squeaking at night. They would joke about what I was doing but I felt less embarrassed by the suggestion that I was frenziedly masturbating than by the fact that I couldn't keep still.

Leftwing Idiot first mentioned my tics shortly after we'd started working together. We were walking back from lunch and he asked, 'Why did your arm just move like that?' I replied, 'It does that sometimes, it has a mind of its own.' He laughed and asked what I meant. I brushed the question off and he said I was strange.

My tics got worse throughout my early twenties and it was generally accepted by my friends that I was pretty twitchy. When Laura and I were working together, each day ended with a lengthy team meeting. During one particularly dull meeting she and our mate Kyle kept a tally of how many silly faces I made. This wasn't something I felt upset about because I knew they weren't being unkind, and I did move about a lot. But I didn't believe they'd counted accurately.

Most people just accepted how I was, though sometimes they found it confusing. Leftwing Idiot found it really weird when, if he asked me what noise dogs make, I would bark. I found it really weird that he could choose not to if he was asked the same thing.

Friends would worry about me in formal situations and would ask if I was able to keep still. Sometimes they'd get annoyed and say, 'You're not trying hard enough to stop.' I sort of agreed. Part of why it took me so long to ask for help was because I kept thinking that if I could just concentrate a bit harder I'd be able to make it stop. But I couldn't, and as the tics increased in complexity and force I felt increasingly frustrated by my lack of control.

I remember wanting to talk to the disability coordinator at college about it. She was providing support for me in other areas and she'd definitely noticed my unusual arm and hand movements, but I bottled out. I talked about it with Laura a couple of times shortly after I started throwing my head back. I told her that when we were out I'd go to the loo and move about wildly. I didn't think this was particularly odd and tried to convince her to give it a try.

It was my mum who first said out loud she thought I had Tourettes. She'd watched a documentary looking at whether Mozart had the condition and thought what it described sounded like me. But I did nothing about it, thinking that if I'd gone this long without a proper diagnosis I didn't need one. But my tics were having an increasing impact on my life, both socially and at work.

One day a friend of mine asked, 'How can I explain your twitching to my friends when you meet them?' This question really stuck in my mind and made me realise it might be time to have a fuller explanation for my behaviour, both for me and for other people. I emailed Leftwing Idiot a link to the symptoms and diagnosis criteria for Tourettes and asked him to have a look. A few minutes later he phoned and said, 'You have Tourettes. Now what are you going to do about it?'

Most people with Tourettes have tics from childhood, but having listened to other people's stories I've realised my experience of not being diagnosed until later isn't that uncommon. I've met several people who, like me, have much more extreme tics as adults than they had when they were younger. It can go the other way too, and for lots of children with Tourettes, their tics won't be a big challenge in adulthood.

My parents always worried about people labelling me when I was a child, but I remember Superman's foster parents having the same dilemma, and I've never regretted seeking help to understand better something that's a big part of my life.

STRONG YOUNG MINDS

There was a large group of teenage boys behind me on the bus this morning. They started laughing at me as soon as they sat down, but I could hear one voice of dissent. Instead of laughing, he was quietly reasoning with his friends, saying things like, 'I don't see what's funny. Imagine if it was your mum or your sister,' and 'You lot are being rude. It could be your family.'

After listening to all this for a few minutes I turned to the group and said, 'I don't know which of you it is, but someone's speaking a lot of sense. Whoever it is, you're very strong to stand up to your mates. Thank you.'

One of the boys reached over to his friend, put his hand on his shoulder and said, 'She's speaking to you.'

DAMAGE LIMITATION

My knuckles are giving in. It might be the cold weather, but the skin has eroded on my hands where I bang them against my chest to a point where they're cracked and bleeding. This skin damage makes banging my chest hundreds of times an hour even more painful. Leftwing Idiot's done a little internet research and found some padded fingerless boxing gloves. They look pretty stylish so I'm going to give them a try.

WAS THAT ME?

While I was out this evening a young man started to mimic the noises I was making. Bizarrely, he was so good at it that to begin with I was unsure whether it was me or not.

Once I'd worked it out I explained to the man that I had Tourettes. He seemed surprised. 'I thought people with Tourettes swore.'

His mate answered, 'It affects everyone differently.'

I confirmed this was true and explained that only 10% of people with Tourettes swear.

But as I walked away I started swearing and I heard the young man say to his friend, 'See? Did you hear that?'

CAN'T STOP

Leftwing Idiot and I were out locally today. I was emitting my normal, frequent, unusual noises. As we walked past a police officer on a bike at the traffic lights she turned towards us, pointed at me and yelled, 'Stop that!' I was surprised by how angry I felt so I turned back to explain. This isn't the first time I've been challenged by the police and they're often ungracious, even after I've explained I have Tourettes. On another occasion a policeman warned me, 'You can't behave like that.'

It's not that simple.

DOPEY, SLEEPY OR JUST SNEEZY?

A couple of days ago I started a new course of medication for Tourettes, but now I'm faced with the tricky decision of whether to go on with it. It's a drug I was on a couple of years ago but I gave it up when it stopped working.

My doctor thought that because things are getting more difficult it was worth trying again, and that it might work better now I've had a break from it. We agreed that I should take it for a few days, stop for a few days, and then start again. The idea was that this pattern might help make the drug work better and reduce the side effects.

I'm having second thoughts now because I've been struggling since I started taking it again. I've felt exhausted, it's been hard to focus, I've had to fight to keep my eyes open and I've found myself suddenly feeling sick a few times.

Of course, I might just be a bit unwell, for reasons completely unrelated to the medication. Even so, I reckon I won't take tonight's dose and see how I feel tomorrow.

FEBRUARY

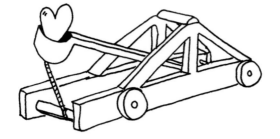

CATAPULT YOUR LOVE TO ME

THE FIRST FUCK

I'm a couple of days into my new job. My boss heard her first 'fuck' today. I think she'd had the impression that I was one of the 90% of people with Tourettes who don't swear. That illusion is now broken.

'Fucking, fucking, fucking, Ginger Rogers.'
'To me, to me, to me, to you, to you, fuck off.'
'The first fuck is the deepest.'

I work for an organisation in South London that runs play projects for children and young people. My role is a mixture of fundraising and development. I've worked with children for years, although my previous jobs have always been at specialist inclusive places. This is the first time I've ever worked for an organisation that doesn't focus specifically on services for disabled children.

You might wonder how anyone who swears involuntarily can possibly work with children.

The key issue with all swearing is the intention behind it, but my swearing is completely involuntary and when I tic 'fuck' it has no more meaning than when I tic 'biscuit'. I reckon children who are old enough to recognise a swear word or ask what it means are also old enough to understand that I've not chosen to swear, and that it isn't OK for them to do it, particularly if it's aimed at someone else.

There are people who would argue that exposing children to bad language is not acceptable because it might confuse them or encourage them to repeat what they hear. I completely disagree and argue that it's entirely appropriate for children to be in environments where difference is accepted, understood and

supported, even if that means putting up with the odd exple-
tive.

The fact is, any swear word that escapes from my mouth does
so in the context of other unusual noises and movements, so it
becomes something that everyone's familiar with.

It's true my tics have increased in intensity since I started
working with children, and had they been as noticeable when I
started I think it would've been much harder for me to develop
the confidence and skills needed to do this work. I've been
incredibly well supported and my colleagues have always shared
the humour Tourettes can bring.

Although I think there are ways for people with Tourettes to
overcome most employment challenges and do jobs people
might think are not compatible with the condition (for example
there's a surgeon with Tourettes), there are some career paths I
wouldn't pursue, especially those involving stillness, silence or
secrecy. I might find being a living statue, sound recordist or spy
too much of a challenge. However, being a superhero is well
within my capability.

THUMP-A-YOUTH MAN

While I was sitting outside a pub tonight with my friend Kyle, a
passing stranger saw me and stopped. 'Oh my God, it's you,' he
said. I'd started rifling through my mind trying to identify him
when he told me, 'I thumped a youth for you the other day.' That
didn't clarify anything.

'You've got Tourettes Syndrome, right? There were some
youths laughing at you on the bus, you got off and I told one of
them not to laugh. He carried on, so I thumped him. Wham!'

A detailed re-enactment of the thumping followed. I told him
I appreciated the sentiment but wasn't entirely sure about the
level of violence.

He carried on, 'You can't laugh, that's not on. Disabilities are cool.' He stepped back to allow a man using a wheelchair to pass. 'They shouldn't laugh like that. You can't help it. It's Tourettes.'

I think Thump-A-Youth Man could see I was surprised, and he reassured me he wouldn't normally do anything like that.

'I got off the bus, walked round the corner and called my missus. I told her what'd happened and started crying. Then she started crying.'

Thump-A-Youth Man let me know he was looking out for me and disappeared into the night.

COUNTING AND SHOUTING

I share an office with two colleagues who, on the whole, barely seem to notice my tics. Today, however, one of them had to move to the room next door because they were too distracting. She was totalling a series of numbers, carefully and quietly counting out loud. I was counting a lot less quietly and much more randomly. 'Forty-eight, sixty-two, I'm four, I'm forty-four, I'm fourteen.'

ODDS

I often underestimate how much I tic, and overestimate my ability to control them.

This evening I made a reckless bet with Leftwing Idiot. I said I'd give him a pound every time I ticced if he gave me a fiver for every tic-free minute. We agreed to cap the bet at five minutes.

I owe him fifty quid.

CURIOUS QUESTIONS ARE FINE

I had an appointment this morning with a doctor who doesn't specialise in Tourettes. At the end of the consultation he said,

'I think that's all the questions I have, except the nosey ones. I haven't seen much Tourettes.' He went on to ask me several questions and also suggested I apply for Disability Living Allowance, which I'd thought I wouldn't be entitled to because I work. He said it wouldn't be a problem so I'll look into it further.

Genuine questions are cool, whoever asks them, and on the whole I'm happy to answer. In fact I'm prone to asking nosey questions myself:

'What are you doing with your life?'
'If you got raped by a biscuit would you tell anyone?'
'Do you want to imagine a bear having sex with a keyboard?'

I thought now might be a good time to get some frequently asked questions out of the way (although I cover more of them in a chapter at the end of this book), so for the rest of this entry I'm going to cover the questions I was asked by a thirty-strong under-11s football team on the top deck of a bus this afternoon:

WHY CAN'T YOU STOP DOING THAT?

I explained to the boys that my brain was making my body move and make noises without my choosing, a bit like blinking or sneezing. This was generally accepted, except by a small boy sitting opposite me. He told me he hadn't sneezed for years.

HOW DO YOU SLEEP?

With difficulty, although on the whole I don't tic when I'm asleep. However, on the occasions when I do wake up shouting, jerking or throwing myself against a wall, it can be quite unsettling.

CAN YOU EAT?

Yes.

WHAT WOULD HAPPEN IF WE TIED YOUR HANDS UP?

I'd be annoyed. I do sometimes sit on my hands or lie with them tucked under my body or head at night. There are some occasions when a friend might hold my hands still. Personally, I find it a big relief when someone I trust takes over for a while. A less welcome intervention occurred once when a stranger at a bus stop grabbed my arms and shouted at me to stop.

WHY DO YOU SAY THOSE WORDS?

I don't have a clue. They're mostly random and not related to specific events or thoughts. Sometimes, however, they're a response to something I've seen or heard.

DO SOME PEOPLE LAUGH AT YOU?

Yes. Sometimes people laugh at me. Sometimes they laugh because I've said something funny. Sometimes I laugh at myself. There's a big difference between laughing at things that are genuinely funny and laughing at somebody because they're moving in a different way or making unusual noises.

COULD IT HAPPEN TO ME?

Several boys asked this in slightly different ways. Although it isn't really known what triggers Tourettes, it affects people from all backgrounds and has been reported the world over. It normally becomes apparent when people are about seven years old, but it can start much later.

At this point, with most of the top deck involved in our impromptu Q&A, another passenger helpfully pointed out to the boys that there was still enough time for it to happen to them.

DO YOU EVER SAY STUFF ON PURPOSE AND PRETEND YOU DIDN'T MEAN TO?

No. I've never claimed something was a tic when it wasn't. Tics tend to sound different to my normal speaking voice, but sometimes I have to make it clear to people when I've actually *chosen* to say something and am expecting a response.

The only other frequently asked question not covered by the junior football team is one I don't usually answer until at least the third date.

SHAMPOO BOWLING

Tourettes can make even the simplest things tricky. This morning I was trying to wash my hair but kept throwing the bottle of shampoo. If bathroom bowling was a recognised sport I would've definitely got a strike – all the other bottles at the end of the bath went flying.

SAFETY FIRST, SECOND AND THIRD

Earlier today I was talking to King Russell. He was in his room and I was standing in the doorway. He called me over, saying, 'Come here a second.' As soon as I was in the room he shut the door behind me and said, 'You were jerking around far too close to the top of the stairs.'

This afternoon I was at Poppy's house. She's a costume designer and often works at home. While I was standing by her desk I absently picked up a big pair of sharp scissors. 'What've you got there?' she asked as she darted across the room to disarm me.

Tonight I was watching a film at Leftwing Idiot's. I was stretched out on the floor and struggling to keep still. He reached out and said, 'Come and sit on the sofa.' I said, 'I'll be fine in a minute', but a minute later I head-butted the floor. He helped me onto the sofa and held me still until I was calmer.

I do try to look after myself but I'd certainly get hurt a lot more if my friends weren't so alert.

THE SAME, THE UGLY AND THE GOOD

I'm going to share thirty minutes of my day through the reactions I've encountered along the way.

3.OOPM

I popped to the shops during my lunch break to pick up some plasters to protect my knuckles from the wear and tear they're currently suffering from all my chest banging. While I was browsing in the chemist, I squawked loudly. There were two young women next to me and one asked the other, 'Was that you?' I looked round at her and said, 'No it was me, I have Tourettes.' She smiled and said, 'So has she', nodding in the direction of her friend. This wasn't the response I was expecting. We chatted for a minute before getting on with our shopping.

3.15PM

When I was walking back to work I saw a middle-aged man coming towards me. I squeaked once as I got near him and when we drew level he shouted a similar noise to the one I'd just made, quite threateningly. I turned and asked, 'Why did you do that?' He responded aggressively, 'I was copying you.' I told him I had Tourettes and that the noise wasn't directed at him. 'I don't care, you can fuck off', he said. He walked off shouting offensive things at me all the way down the street. I got back to work feeling shaken and angry.

3.3OPM

After I'd had a chat with my colleagues about what had happened, I spent some time with the children I work with who were playing on the computer and dashing in and out of the building. While I was putting the plasters on my knuckles a few of the younger boys asked me what I was doing. I explained that I was protecting the skin on my hand because it was getting sore from where I banged my chest. One of the boys asked, 'Why do you bang your chest?' The youngest boy, whom I'd met for the first time a couple of days before, answered for me: 'Her brain makes her do it, it controls her arm.' He paused briefly, and added, 'and her mouth.'

When I started my new job I'd explained to the children why I sometimes make unusual noises and movements. It's great when they start to answer each other's questions in their own words, and hearing this child explain it so straightforwardly reassured me that my answers to their questions had been clear enough and were fully understood.

These three accounts illustrate the varied reactions my tics provoke. I never know how people will react. There's not one group or type of person that seems to respond more positively or negatively than any other. All I know is, when I leave my house in the morning other people *will* react, and their reactions *will* be mixed. I'm sure this isn't unique to Tourettes, but is something that's experienced by people with any conditions that make them stand out.

I'M IN LOVE

Poppy's made me the most amazing gift ever. I'm now the very proud owner of a pair of bespoke padded gloves that are light, beautiful, stylish, comfortable and above all not red.

Don't get me wrong. I like red as much as anyone else, but for the last month I've been wearing the same red woollen boxing mitts to protect hands, chest and face from ferocious and frequent arm tics. There's no doubt they've saved me from a great deal of pain. But I was desperate for a new colour and Poppy's new pair has surpassed all my expectations.

I think I'm a little bit in love with my own hands.

MOVING ON

When I started writing this diary, I resolved to be honest but not to slip into self-pity. Tonight, in this entry, I'm going to tread that fine line – I've been feeling overwhelmingly upset all day.

It was a conversation with an elderly woman on a bus that started it off. I don't write about every negative exchange but I've decided to describe this one because I suspect there are many people who think about Tourettes in a similar way.

I sat down next to the woman and she started tutting and sighing whenever I ticced.

TH: If I'm swearing it's not at you or because I'm rude, it's because I have Tourettes Syndrome and I can't control the movements and noises I make.

Woman: You *are* rude and you keep swearing.

TH: I can't control it; I'm not choosing to swear.

Woman: I don't believe in Tourettes.

TH: I wish I could 'not believe' in Tourettes too, but that's not really an option for me.

Woman: You just need to stop it. Why is it only bad words?

TH: It's not only swear words. You can hear that I also say 'biscuit' and lots of other words.

Woman: I'm not interested in the other words. You should stop being offensive.

TH: I'm not saying offensive words deliberately. They aren't directed at anyone and they don't mean anything.

Woman: Look at the children over there, they have to listen to you. What do you think *they* think?

TH: I hope they can see a woman who makes a lot of different noises and movements she clearly can't control, but also someone who's able to have a thoughtful conversation.

Woman: How do those bad words get into your head? You must be bad or someone must have put them there.

TH: *You* know swear words too, but can choose not to say them. *I* can't stop any word I know from turning into a tic that I keep repeating.

Woman: Rubbish! You should stop. I don't think you're even *trying* to stop. You should just stop saying the swear words. I don't care about 'biscuit'.

At this point a passenger sitting behind us interjected.

Passenger Two: If I can give you a doctor's opinion, what you're asking her to do isn't possible. She has Tourettes Syndrome, which means the connections in her brain aren't working properly and she can't stop the noises she makes.

Woman: Why is it bad words? Someone must have put them in her head.

Passenger Two: As she explained, it's a mix of noises.

A third passenger standing nearby then spoke to the woman.

Passenger Three: Don't worry about her. I don't think she's very well.

TH: I'm not sick. I just have a condition that means I make noises and movements I can't control. But I *am* in control of my thoughts.

My stop was coming up and with relief I thanked the doctor, said goodbye to both women and got off the bus. As I walked away I felt shaky and tearful but managed to compose myself.

Later, at Leftwing Idiot's, we talked about what'd happened while he was making dinner. He told me not to dwell on it, but suddenly, from nowhere, I started to cry uncontrollably. I felt drained by the relentlessness of my tics, by the constant need to explain them, by the judgements of other people, and by feeling humiliated so frequently. When I stopped crying and started to feel better, Leftwing Idiot pointed out that I didn't need to worry about any of that in his house. He said he knew how difficult things have been getting for me recently. His empathy and reassurance helped me let it go.

TODDLERS LOVE TICS

This afternoon I hung out with my friend Gurpreet and her two-and-a-half-year-old son Owain.

Owain loves Tourettes. He laughs, joins in and says, 'Again!' after every tic. Owain's enjoyment of my tics is the most joyful reaction I've ever experienced. He particularly loves the biscuits. Owain isn't a passive observer either – he jumps in, getting his squeak on and flapping about.

I had a lovely afternoon and I'm pretty sure he did too.

MIND OVER MUSCLE

A few weeks ago I started Habit Reversal Therapy (HRT). This is an approach to managing tics that uses very specific behavioural techniques. It aims to teach you to replace damaging tics with ones that have less physical or social impact. I'd been keen to try this option since I first heard about it a while back because my tics have been getting worse and I'm injuring myself frequently as a result.

This afternoon I went for another session. I've found the last couple of weeks of HRT difficult, not because of anything I'm being asked to do physically, but because of how it challenges the way I think about my tics.

I felt particularly confused after a session last week during which we'd been exploring the way thoughts and emotions might influence tics. While I know that both have a noticeable effect, I've always felt strongly that they're not the root cause.

While we were talking, the therapist said he'd not seen any

evidence that Tourettes was neurological. I pointed out that there's also no evidence that it's anything other than neurological, and that there's a frustrating lack of research into Tourettes generally.

It's taken a long time for me to get to a point where I can accept my tics and not blame myself for having them. But after I left the appointment last week I felt as though this had been undermined, and each time I ticced I felt disgusted with myself.

I know this wasn't the therapist's intention and that he hadn't been suggesting I could just stop ticcing. But perhaps because I often look like a stereotypical 'mad woman', I'm very sensitive about theories that suggest tics are caused by psychological factors.

The fact is, I don't live with Tourettes as a theory. I live with the relentless movement, noise and unusual experiences it brings. To maintain my sanity and self-confidence I hang on to the fact that I *do* have control over my thoughts and feelings, even if I can't always control my body or speech.

When I got home after last week's session I talked to Fat Sister about how it'd made me feel. She said she thinks Tourettes is multi-factorial, meaning there's a mix of different issues involved – neurological as well as emotional and behavioural. This makes a lot of sense to me.

For a long time I worked as part of a team that helped children with autism. It's generally accepted that autism is purely neurological, even though there's little hard evidence to support this. It's also clear that behavioural techniques can play a major part in its treatment. But this obviously doesn't make it a psychological condition. It's just what seems to work best.

I've been thinking about the psychological aspect of my tics all week and it's upset and confused me. We talked about it again at my appointment today, and afterwards, on my way home, I realised it doesn't matter to me at all what actually causes my tics.

Different theories about what makes me tic aren't that important. What does matter is that I keep an open mind about all the possible methods of dealing with Tourettes, and if I try them, I do so wholeheartedly.

TUBES, TERROR AND TICCING

It's been a while since I've travelled by tube at rush hour. It's a pretty unpleasant experience for everyone, and this evening I experienced the added difficulties that having Tourettes can present in this situation.

I waited on a busy platform at Green Park, squawking, jerking and shouting. The challenge of tube travel at this time of day is to stand at the edge of the platform right where the train doors will open to get a space on the train. This task isn't compatible with unpredictable, uncontrollable jerking.

I had to keep retreating to the back of the platform and content myself with shouting helpful instructions like 'Push!' and responding to security announcements by shouting 'Bomb, bomb, bang!' I also contributed some less relevant instructions – 'Piano practice now!'

Seven packed trains went through before I was eventually able to get on one. My frustration was compounded by the fact that I was meeting Laura for dinner, and she was quite likely to have wilted away with hunger while I battled to secure a safe spot under someone's armpit.

MARCH

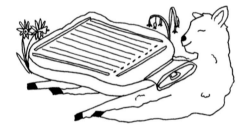

GOODNIGHT   WINTER   I KNOW
THERE'S   A   SPRING   UNDERNEATH YOU.

THE 230-MILLION-YEAR-OLD BEAST IN MY BELLY

Today I have been mostly channelling dinosaurs. As well as shouting about biscuits and waving my arms around, I'm in the process of adding various different prehistoric screeches to my collection of tics. It sounds like I've just got stuck in Tourassic Park.

Physical tics – known to the medical profession as motor tics – are difficult to describe but are as much a part of my life with Tourettes as the things I say. I make these movements all day and they include:

Banging my chest with my fist (it's as painful as it sounds)
Jerking my head backwards
Blinking and grimacing
Bending my wrists and elbows sharply
Stamping my feet and bending my knees
Rising suddenly onto my toes

Physical tics make completing even small tasks difficult. For instance, turning on a light switch or putting my debit card in a cash machine can prove tricky. I find physical tics more distressing than vocal tics, but I've always thought if I had the choice to get rid of them or the noises, I'd choose the vocal tics because I've always thought they were more intrusive.

However, I was chatting about this with Leftwing Idiot the other day and he said he found the physical tics more troubling because I look so uncomfortable. Physical tics have a strong sensation attached to them – it's intense, uncomfortable and impossible to ignore. It feels like it's coming from deep inside my body, and it isn't always located in the area where the actual tic

occurs. For instance, when I hit my chest, the feeling I'm responding to is often located in the middle of my back. But the presence
of the sensation doesn't usually mean I know a tic's about to
happen – my body responds instinctively, and I only realise I'm
ticcing after it's happened.

Sometimes I can catch myself halfway through a tic. If I really
concentrate and shut down the rest of me, I can keep still for very
short periods of time, much like how you can stop yourself blinking if you try hard enough.

IN THE FACE OF LAUGHTER

When I'm out and about on my own, strangers tend to react differently to me from when I'm with friends, but this isn't because
of any change in me or my tics. When the unusual noises and
movements I make are interspersed with clearly *normal* conversations, other people are less likely to be afraid of me because
they can see and hear I'm not *mad* and will know if they're talking about me.

Tonight I travelled home with Leftwing Idiot on a bus. It was
busy and I sat down as soon as a seat became available. Leftwing
Idiot stayed standing nearby – close, but not close enough for us
to have a conversation.

A man got on at the next stop and I knew immediately he was
going to say something to me. He was behaving erratically him-
self, and when he spotted me he started to copy the noises I was
making, loudly and very inaccurately.

He stopped in front of me and continued the mockery. I said,
'Yes, I'm making some noises and it'll keep happening.' He started
copying my chest banging, and then he reached out and banged
my chest! I said, 'Don't do that, it's bad enough that I do it to
myself.' He told me he was a good fighter, and I said, 'That's
great – I don't need you to show me though.' He looked at me
and said, 'You're safe; I'm mad but you're OK.'

Leftwing Idiot didn't interfere during this exchange. I think if he had, things could have escalated. And I'm used to managing situations like this on my own. Occasionally people I don't know get involved, sometimes brilliantly, sometimes chaotically.

Three recent examples that all occurred on buses spring to mind:

POWERFUL, PEACEFUL, POLITE

A group of six or seven teenage girls were laughing at me. I challenged them but they continued so I ignored them. I was aware during this uncomfortable journey that one of the girls was not laughing or joining in, and I heard her say, 'I don't see what's funny.' When they got up to leave she stopped and said, 'I'm really sorry for my friends' behaviour, I hope you have a nice day.'

SHAMING THE IGNORANT

A mother and her son were sitting next to me. There were some older men sitting behind me who were laughing at me and making comments. I acknowledged them but as I'd already challenged someone else on the same bus I didn't really feel like doing it again. The woman next to me turned to them and said, 'I've just explained to my son why it's not right to laugh. He's a child – why don't you know better?'

A FORCEFUL STOP IT

I'd been in town and was travelling back on a busy bus with a couple sitting behind me. I said something funny and complicated about squirrels and heard the man giggle. Shortly afterwards a group of tourists got on. One of them went to sit down next to me and I squeaked. She stopped so I said, 'It's OK. It's fine to sit here." She took no notice and stared at me blankly for a few moments before moving away. A couple of her friends sat opposite me, laughing relentlessly and exchanging comments. I didn't know what language they were speaking so I wasn't sure if their laughter was directed at me, although it got louder when I ticced which gave me the impression I was the cause of their escalating hilarity.

Eventually the man with his girlfriend got annoyed and said to the group, 'Stop laughing at her.' The woman who'd ignored me said, 'We're not laughing at her and it's not your business.' The man replied, 'You are, and it's rude.' He turned back and I thanked him.

Laughter's a common reaction, and I understand Tourettes might look funny if you've not encountered it before. Strangely, I find people laughing at me or having overtly hostile reactions the easiest to deal with. Staring, tutting or frightened and disgusted looks are much more difficult because I don't know when to say something. I'm not oversensitive and only challenge disrespect-ful behaviour that I'm sure is related to me.

The laughing tourists were lucky Thump-A-Youth Man wasn't there.

PARENTAL APPROACH

I was at a cash point this evening doing my best to get some money out. A mother and her two children came and stood behind me in the queue; they were chatting happily about where to go for an after-school snack.

Both the children looked at me with curiosity. I smiled at them and the younger child smiled back, but his sister looked nerv-ously at her mum and said, 'Why does that woman keep moving?' Her mother didn't respond. The girl persisted, but she still ignored the question.

I decided to explain and told her that my brain sometimes makes me move and make noises I can't control. I reassured her it was nothing to worry about and the girl seemed to relax a bit. Her brother smiled cheerfully, but their mother looked anxious and didn't say anything to me, or even look at me.

While some adults find children's questions about Tourettes

uncomfortable, I don't. Neither do some parents, and I've got a lot of respect for adults who overcome their own self-consciousness to make sure their children understand whatever's puzzling them.

Once I was on a bus and a mother got on with her daughter. The mum looked round a few times before saying to me, 'Sorry, but I need to ask, what's wrong with you? My daughter's asking and I want to give her the right information.' And this gave me the opportunity to explain.

One of my favourite explanations came from a father whose son was pointing at me and saying, 'That lady's being silly.' He said, 'She's not silly, she's expressing herself.'

DIRECT ACTION

My Tourettes Syndrome public relations campaign continues.

This morning I offered my seat to an elderly man, picked up a woman's spilt shopping and cooed/squeaked over a newborn baby.

I often feel the need to make an extra effort to make my actions speak louder than my words to demonstrate that, despite my flapping arms and odd language, I'm not rude.

I like to think I'd do these sorts of things just as often if I didn't have Tourettes. But I know that having positive interactions with strangers is a way of challenging the judgements they might make about me. They can also lead to great conversations. I'm off to open some doors.

JIM DOESN'T FIX IT FOR MOST PEOPLE

My tics fall into three broad categories. First, the regular tics I say hundreds of times every day. Second, the occasional tics that I'll say just once (or a handful of times). I've already discussed these two categories, but I haven't yet talked about the third type.

These are intense explosions of themed tics that come out over a short period of time with incredible force. They're sometimes triggered by hearing or seeing something specific, but often occur for no apparent reason. These outbursts are unpredictable and only happen every couple of months. They can last from ten minutes to a few hours and are so overwhelming it's hard to do or say anything else while they're flying out.

During these explosive sessions a number of different tics will come out that are linked by a theme, tune or sound. When it eventually stops, one or two of these tics might hang around and become regulars. I'm currently saying, 'Biscuit, biscuit, biscuit bear,' which is a remnant of one such episode.

Tonight I had one of these explosive events after I inadvertently heard the opening bars of the *Jim'll Fix It* theme tune. For international readers, and those born after 1990, this was a TV programme featuring a sinister old man in a tracksuit making wishes come true for his hopeful young viewers. The man in question is now dead.

Hearing this long-forgotten theme tune sparked an involuntary reworking of the lyrics that I repeated continuously over the next two hours. It went something like this:

'One letter is only the start of it – badly written.'
'One letter – and then he wanks on your shoe.'
'One letter – never answered.'
'Grooming!'
'One letter – and then the bailiffs know where you live.'
'One letter is only the start of it – possible rape victim.'
'And you, and you, and ba, ba, baa.'

'Jim'll fix it – if you're pretty.'
'Jim'll fix it – if you're vulnerable.'
'Jim'll fix it – if you're parents don't care enough to save you.'
'Jim doesn't fix it for most people.'
'Not you or you or ba, ba, baa.'

The power of certain sounds is something I don't understand, and some days I seem more sensitive to the things I hear than others. I suspect this is linked to echolalia, a fairly common feature of Tourettes and other neurological conditions, which involves repeating noises or phrases made by other people. It's got me into trouble before now, when strangers have thought I'm taking the piss.

Dear Jim, can you forgive me?

UNKIND ACT

This isn't going to be what I'd planned to write.

I've unexpectedly been left feeling sad and undermined by something that happened earlier. I'd had a great evening with Laura and was coming home on the bus. Just as I was getting off, and too late for me to respond, a man sitting near the door said, 'You're a good actor.'

I'm used to being judged by strangers and obviously I shouldn't dwell on a comment made by someone I don't know, but what this man said left me feeling dented.

I couldn't work out why I felt so hurt at first, but then I realised what upset me wasn't that he'd judged my behaviour, but that he'd judged my character by suggesting I was just pretending.

PARROT

King Russell's mum called earlier and while he was speaking to her I was squawking away in the background as usual. Then I heard him say, 'No mum, we haven't bought a parrot.' He went on to explain it was just me she could hear shrieking.

King Russell's mum knows me well but she hadn't heard this particular squawk before. Sometimes I *am* like a parrot and do repeat things I've just heard.

JUST IMPEDIMENT

This morning, Fat Sister and King Russell went to our local registry office to declare formally their intent to marry, and set a date in June.

When one of Fat Sister's friends heard the news she made a joke about shouting out inappropriate things during the ceremony. Fat Sister said, 'You do realise my sister's going to be there? Do you really think you can compete with her?'

We shall see.

MADNESS AND ME

I've already talked a bit about the psychological factors that influence Tourettes. Thinking about mental health in greater depth has exposed some of my own archaic attitudes to the subject. For example I find it hard to shake off the idea there's shame involved in having a mental health 'problem'.

I talk a lot about madness but never actually give my own mental wellbeing much thought because I find it too uncomfortable. When I'm struggling with my tics I often seek reassurance from those around me and ask them, 'Am I mad?'

Two key things seem to fuel my awkward relationship with madness. The first is that strangers often treat me like I'm crazy. Because of how my tics look, they assume I'm mentally unwell and sometimes respond with fear. This reinforces my own negative attitudes and feeds a constant need to prove I'm 'sane'.

The second is that my strange behaviour makes *me* feel I'm crazy. I do things that confuse and frighten me, like biting my hand or running into the road. These things don't scare me because of their inherent riskiness but because I don't understand where the behaviour comes from.

Some friends describe me as the sanest person they know, and this always feels like winning a massive prize. But it's the importance I place on the opinions of others that's probably the strangest aspect of the way I think.

I talked to Leftwing Idiot about all this and he said, 'The only thing that ever feels close to a mental health issue with you is your concern about what other people think. But it's not that straightforward because some people *do* judge you.'

He's right. Recently I overheard a man on the bus say, 'Look at that psychiatric patient over there.' He was of course pointing at me.

The importance I place on how I'm perceived isn't very healthy. Alongside using Habit Reversal Therapy to help regain control of my movements, I'm going to work on improving my emotional balance, and on taking greater care of my mental wellbeing. Wish me luck.

MYSTERIOUS

Yesterday I ticced, throwing my head back and hitting it against the wall. 'Mystery.'

This morning I twisted my ankle with a strange leg tic. 'Mystery.'

And I hit myself in the face. 'Mystery.'

Tonight I banged my hand on a shelf in a shop. 'Mystery.'

And just now when I thumped my chin, Leftwing Idiot and I said in unison: 'Mystery.'

'I always know when you've hurt yourself,' he said, 'because you say "Mystery".'

It would seem 'Ouch' just won't do any more.

DRUMMING LESSONS

It's been a full-on day. A summary would look a bit like this:

Travelling, laughing, banging, confronting, sobbing, regrouping, eating, reflecting, relaxing.

But I suppose I should put in a bit more detail, so here goes.

Ruth and I travelled to Sheffield for a drumming workshop for people with Tourettes. On the train we were chatting, laughing and enjoying each other's company. Then a woman claiming to be a go-between for Jesus came and spoke to us. She knelt down next to our seats and said that He loved us and wanted to give us a lovely gift. She asked whether there was anything either of us wanted. We politely said there wasn't and declined His help.

The workshop was great, although initially I found it hard to persuade my arms to cooperate and hit the drums rather than myself. I used drum brushes instead of hard sticks, which meant I could concentrate on making a load of noise without worrying about hurting myself.

The journey back wasn't quite as smooth. First, while we were waiting for the train a drunk man took offence because he thought I'd sworn at him. I explained, but he wasn't really in a condition to take it on board. His main concern was that Ruth and I were going to jump in front of a train and delay his journey. We didn't.

When we got on the train Ruth and I had to sit about ten rows apart. This made the noise we were making spread further than if we'd been sitting together. I could hear lots of people around us laughing, but I wasn't too fazed by this. What did upset me was looking up to find that the woman in front of me had pressed her phone between the seats and was filming me. I asked what she was doing and she pulled the phone away without say anything. I asked again, but still no answer. In the end I got up and went to speak to her. I made her delete the video. For the rest of the journey I could see that she was writing down my tics in a notebook.

After Ruth and I said goodbye I went down to catch a tube. While I was waiting on the platform an elderly woman walked past with some friends. She looked at me with disgust and said, 'Eurgh, we have to put up with this, do we?' I said, 'That's not very friendly.' She replied, 'It wasn't meant to be.' I asked her why she was being deliberately nasty, but she ignored me and walked away.

I felt broken, desperately alone and sad. I got on the next tube, really wanting someone to speak to. I thought about reaching out to someone in the carriage, but instead I sat and fought back the tears. I've never cried on public transport before but the woman's comment had really hurt. She could carry on with her day and never be disturbed by my tics again. I don't have that choice.

I held it together on the tube but when I got out I began crying uncontrollably. I called Fat Sister and Laura but neither answered so I phoned King Russell. I willed him to answer and when he finally did he talked to me gently and helped me calm down enough to get on the bus home.

After we'd hung up, a woman sitting near me on the bus who'd heard the conversation leaned forward and asked, 'Would it help if you had someone to talk to?' I said yes, and thanked her. We chatted for the last few minutes of the journey and it helped remind me that more people are understanding and supportive than are thoughtless and unkind.

When I reached the lair a delicious roast dinner was waiting for me. As I ate I thought how great it had been to spend time with Ruth, and then, tired out, I sank into the sofa and began to relax.

I LOVE BYE BYES

This afternoon I went for more Habit Reversal Therapy (HRT). This treatment's helped me feel a lot more in control of my body as well as my thoughts and emotions. I've learnt strategies that have made everyday tasks like eating or brushing my teeth easier.

At today's session we discussed my progress as well as the things I'm still finding difficult, including some problems I'm having with getting around. HRT focuses on the awareness of the sensation that accompanies tics so you can catch them before they happen and do an alternative movement. We agreed that although I've made significant progress in being able to work around my tics, my awareness of them before they happen hasn't changed.

The main problem is that, because I have so many tics and they happen all the time, identifying the sensation of each one is like trying to pick out an individual ant in an anthill. But even if I haven't been able to make much progress with this yet, I *have* become much better at regaining control after I tic.

My therapist can see these improvements too. I'm happy with the progress I've made and feel much better equipped to meet the challenges that remain. We're going to meet much less frequently from now on as I approach the end of the treatment.

BEST FOOT OVER

My tics have started interfering with the way I walk – they're making every step a little more unpredictable. Turning my ankle is one of the most painful new tics. This happens to most people every now and again, but for me it's begun happening many times a day and means I lurch about even more than normal.

Other similar tics include going up onto my toes, kicking and bending my legs, and dropping suddenly to the floor. These are accompanied by some equally erratic arm and head movements, all of which make walking anywhere with me a dramatic affair.

I had to do quite a bit of walking around today and didn't have anyone to hold onto. It made me realise just how difficult and tiring getting about without help's become recently.

APRIL

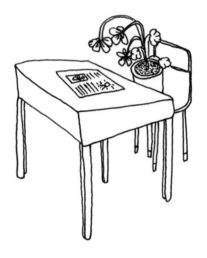

TEACH A GERANIUM ABOUT ITS HISTORY
AND WHY IT'S WORTHLESS.

1:00AM

It's 1am and I'm writing this in bed on my phone. It's a struggle to write because I'm moving so much. I'm exhausted, can't sleep because I keep making a loud howling noise, and my body's contorting all over the place.

I'm trying to stay positive but when things are like this – particularly at night – it can be difficult for me to manage on my own. It's an intense and unpleasant feeling, caused as much by the time of night as by the tics themselves. Thankfully, nights like this don't happen very often.

A QUESTION OF BISCUITS

It's the Easter holidays, which means we're super busy at work. So far the weather's been gorgeous and the playground's full of children enjoying the first sunny spell of the year.

This means there are lots of new children who aren't familiar with me and my tics, so I've spent a lot of time explaining why I say 'biscuit' and bang my chest. They're only being curious and I try to explain Tourettes to them in a way they can understand.

But some of the children who've been there for a while aren't being very patient with the barrage of questions from the new kids. While I was coordinating the creation of a mini-town in the sandpit this afternoon a boy kept asking about my tics until a girl who plays there all the time said to him, 'She's already explained why she says "biscuits" – use your brain or think of a new question!'

Some of the younger children are clearly finding my explanation a little confusing – I overheard one boy explain to another that biscuits had damaged my brain.

Despite this biscuity brain-damage I've managed to have loads of lovely conversations about all sorts of things: Tourettes, dinosaurs, disability, sewage systems, daddy longlegs and the best way to make a swimming pool. It's been a great start to the week.

MISSING IN ACTION

While I was at the playground on Friday afternoon, I took my gloves off to do some washing up. When I turned round one glove had vanished.

This morning I was on the gate, greeting children as they came in for the second week of their Easter holidays. A boy of about six came in and immediately said to me, 'I took your glove last week.'

I asked him why he'd taken it and he said, 'So I could pretend to be you and say "biscuit".'

I explained why I wore the gloves and how without them my hands got sore, and I made sure he understood that taking things without asking was wrong. He's promised to return the missing glove tomorrow.

THE SECOND COMING

A few years ago I went through a big phase of ticcing about God – they were the first tics I responded to creatively. Suddenly, this afternoon while I was sorting out my washing, a fresh batch of 'God' tics burst out. Thank God Poppy jotted down as many as she did:

God said, 'It's a good job I made ketamine for you.'
God said, 'I made skittles for Barking not Dagenham.'
God said, 'It's a good job I made you a foreskin.'

God said, 'Don't worry, it's an iceberg lettuce not a hailstorm.'
God said, 'Don't worry, I'm not going to keep Buckinghamshire.'
God said, 'Noah, learn to swim.'
God said, 'Noah, leave the barn owls behind.'
God said, 'I fucked up with alligators.'
God said, 'I love ashtrays.'
God said, 'I made a seasonal erection a permanent thing.'
God said, 'Magnesium is overrated.'
God said, 'I'd never have invented Spam.'
God said, 'I'm just putting it in your head for now, I'll take it away later.'

The tics stopped as suddenly as they'd started, and I carried on folding my washing.

HOLDING IT TOGETHER

I had a great evening out last night. I caught up with friends I hadn't seen for a while and met lots of new people. Sometimes I worry my personality might get lost under all the wild tics when I meet people for the first time.

Vocal tics have a habit of dominating conversations. New people often ask questions about Tourettes that I'm happy to answer, but it can get boring for friends who've heard it all before.

I find physical tics the hardest to manage though. I don't want my friends to have to hold my hands to stop me hitting myself. I hate it that sometimes I need to be pinned down on the night bus or that couples can't hold hands because they're holding mine. I tried to handle my tics on my own last night but I thumped myself on the nose so hard I felt tears well up.

I'm lucky that one of my biggest concerns is about my friends and the help they so willingly provide. Without that, I'd never be able to go out safely and have a laugh.

OUR AMAZING NHS

Today didn't go as planned.

Thankfully, sixty-three years ago Sir William Beveridge's vision for a national health service became a reality, and it was the NHS that came to my rescue today.

On my way to work I hurt my leg badly when it suddenly ticced at the bottom of the stairs. Even though Leftwing Idiot was holding onto me and I didn't fall far, I landed heavily on my foot and twisted my ankle. There was a horrible loud crunch followed by me shouting 'Mystery' a lot. It was incredibly painful and I knew immediately I wasn't going to be able to ignore it.

Leftwing Idiot was fantastic and calm. We called a cab to take us to hospital, and sat at the bottom of the stairs until it arrived.

From the moment we got there until the moment we left I was treated efficiently, with kindness and understanding.

The taxi pulled up outside A&E. Leftwing Idiot went inside and within seconds reappeared with a porter and a wheelchair. I was wheeled into reception where I gave my details, and a few minutes later a triage nurse saw me. She showed me great empathy and took me to a cubicle where my ankle was examined immediately.

Within twenty minutes of arriving I was on my way to be x-rayed. The radiographers were incredibly cheerful and resourceful in getting clear pictures of my leg despite my tics.

After a short wait a doctor came and told me my ankle wasn't broken and that I could go. But after seeing me trying to walk, he reversed his decision and said it wasn't safe for me to leave because my leg tics were sure to cause further injury. He decided a physio should see me to look at what could be done to help prevent further damage.

I was taken to the clinical decisions unit (CDU). On the way I kept ticcing threats to jump out of the wheelchair so the nurse made sure Leftwing Idiot walked in front to stop me if I did.

No one batted an eyelid at my tics in the CDU and I could see the kindness I was being shown was normal, not exceptional. The physio listened attentively as she assessed me, and took a great deal of care to make sure I was safe to go home. She gave me a big boot to help stabilise the damaged limb, and arranged a follow-up appointment in a few days.

My day had suddenly gone from familiar and routine to frightening and painful, but the NHS was there, as it always is at times of crisis, to provide the help and care I needed. I was reassured and cared for brilliantly throughout and didn't have to complete a single form or discuss any payment plans. The decisions being made were based solely on what I needed – everything was provided quickly, and with good humour.

Obviously a system of this size will not always work perfectly for everyone, but my experience today, and on many other occasions, has reinforced my belief that we need to do everything we can to protect the NHS.

The NHS is under threat. If we can't prevent it, the NHS will stop being the universal, comprehensive public service that looked after me today, and will instead be eaten away by private health care companies. The consequences of losing this amazing service would be devastating for everyone.

IN CELEBRATION

I've been feeling fed up about my tics over the last few days so I've decided to remind myself why they make me a superhero by looking back and choosing my personal top tics.

Reading through the vast collection was enjoyable but I found it hard to pick favourites because so many are entwined with memories of particular times, places or people.

That said, here are some I'm particularly fond of:

'Capital letters talk to themselves at night.'
'Stationary action now.'
'Fingers on buzzards.'
'Don't make me ladder your tights.'
'Night knight riding fish.'
'Hands up Action Man.'
'Raggedy pants.'
'I'm sorry for crashing my life into yours.'

I like these for what they are, but also for what they evoke.

SUGAR-COATED SISTER AND A DEAR DEPARTED DOG

Fat Sister and I had dinner with our mother this evening. I knew none of my more offensive tics would be a problem because she's heard them all before, but her seventeen-year-old dog died last week and I wasn't sure she'd be emotionally ready for my new tic, 'Mummy killed the dog.'

As it turned out, she coped well and no tears were shed – other than tears of laughter when I threw sugar down Fat Sister's top and shouted, 'Sweet tits!'

TALKING TO PLANTS

Fat Sister and King Russell are having a joint hen and stag do which has become known as the hag-do. Twenty-five of us are going to Cornwall tomorrow for four days of camping in tipis. It's not ideal that I've got a twisted ankle and a giant boot on one foot but I'm not going to let that get in the way of a good time.

Many of those coming from outside London are staying at the lair tonight, so I'm staying in Leftwing Idiot's spare room. Shortly after I arrived I was sitting in the kitchen with him and Poppy when I suddenly stuck my fingers up at a newly arrived plant on his kitchen table and shouted: 'Fuck off geranium!'

I don't know why this plant became the target for my tics but it didn't seem upset by them so I carried on into the evening.

HAG-DO DAY ONE -- TRAVELLING AND TIPIS

This morning I woke up with the early-morning sun flooding through the window of Leftwing Idiot's spare room. The view from this window is one of my favourites in London.

Full of anticipation, I walked back to the lair with help from Poppy and Leftwing Idiot. When we got there many more friends had already arrived. Soon we were on the road in four cars heading for the Cornish hag-do. Leftwing Idiot, Poppy and I were in one with King Russell driving. Three further cars were already on the road from other parts of the country. As we got going Leftwing Idiot urged King Russell to get a move on and it quickly became apparent they were treating the journey as a race.

Some people might think a five-hour car journey with someone who has Tourettes would be a nightmare, but my travelling companions seemed to feel the opposite and we had a laugh on the journey with my tics making some interesting contributions.

Here's how we passed the time:

Tourettes MCing to 90s UK garage
I Spy (always a challenge with Tourettes)
Tourettes singalong
Spontaneous horoscopes
One-word-at-a-time stories
Tourettes sat nav

Interspersed with:

'Shall we have a quiet moment for donkeys?'
'I'm just going to sit and stroke a donkey until it says biscuit.'
'I'm partially an eclipse.'
'The beast of Bodmin might be me.'

Despite not having the best or fastest car, we reached the tipi village before everyone else.

The campsite's absolutely stunning, the tipis are spacious and light and I'm excited about the next few days in this gorgeous place.

HAG-DO DAY TWO -- AN AWESOME SPEECH

I stepped out of the tipi this morning into the beautiful green clearing. It was already busy with everyone waking up and preparing for the day. King Russell's brother Carl was sorting out last-minute arrangements for the humiliation of his sibling at the separate stag activities due later in the day. I got busy making sure everything was ready for our hen plans too.

After breakfast we all went to the nearby town of Padstow, where the stags and hens split up. The stags took King Russell, dressed up as a Viking, out on a fishing boat to catch some dinner. The sea was distinctly choppy and many of them came back looking pretty sick.

We hens stayed on dry land and went for lunch at a famous fish café. After we'd eaten, the other hens drifted out of the restaurant bit by bit until just Fat Sister and I were left. I then gave her the first clue to a treasure hunt in which she had to find all the others. She was completely over-excited by this and squealed with glee. Fat Sister shows no sign that she comes from a gene pool enriched by Tourettes except when she's really excited. Then she claps and flaps uncontrollably like a performing seal. It took her a minute to calm down enough to concentrate on the clue.

The treasure hunt ended in a traditional tearoom where we had a cream tea with freshly made scones. Fat Sister got given a treasure box full of envelopes containing messages and photos from each of us. We rejoined the boys and headed back to the campsite.

At the tipis I went with a few of the others for a swim in the lake. As I limped off the pontoon and landed in the deep and freezing water I thought, 'Uh oh! Come on body, you've really got to do as I say now.' I made it safely if noisily to the other pontoon. After drying off we set about the night's celebrations.

Fat Sister and King Russell had made it very clear that what they most wanted from the weekend was a big party with their friends, in a forest. This is exactly what they got. Everyone dressed up in formal evening wear and we had a forest cocktail party.

Much later, when we were all sitting around the fire, Fat Sister gave a long drunken speech in which she talked about and thanked each person in turn. After a while her rambling monologue ran out of steam and she started pointing at people in turn, saying, 'You're awesome, and you're awesome, and you're awesome!'

This won't be forgotten quickly and I'm fairly certain it'll come up again in the wedding speeches, not least because I'll be making one of them.

HAG-DO DAY THREE -- DUCK OFF

After a lazy start to the morning, pretty much all of us headed to the beach. It was a gorgeous clear day and we wanted to make the most of it. After we'd had a paddle, Leftwing Idiot, Poppy and I left the others relaxing on the sand and went to get chips and ice cream.

We ate our cheesy chips sitting next to a canal that runs through the Cornish town of Bude. There were some ducks on the water and my tics gave them the same hostile treatment I gave the geranium the other day:

> *TH*: Fuck off ducks.
> *Leftwing Idiot*: What did they do to deserve that?
> *TH*: Failures.
> *Leftwing Idiot*: How?
> *TH*: Failed pterodactyls.

Evolution's a total mystery to me but I'm reasonably sure this isn't accurate.

POST ZEN OUT

A woman started screaming at me in the post office this afternoon. I explained I had Tourettes but she carried on shouting at me to stop swearing.

I felt upset for a moment but I suddenly realised there was nothing more I could do and there was no point in worrying about it. I felt my body relax and I ignored her. She continued to complain loudly about me until a member of staff shouted at her to stop.

I felt amazingly calm as I walked back to the lair. I thought about how brilliant it had been at the hag-do not having to think about other people's reactions at all. Being in a place where everyone understood, I'd been able to get on with things, and be myself without having to give an explanation.

I'm not sad it's over, though. I just feel lucky to have had the chance to hang out with great friends, and pleased it's shown me I'm not getting 'lost under my tics' as I've sometimes feared.

BIG SECRETS, GOOD NEWS

I went for a drink with Laura and Emma this evening. Laura's pregnant and although I've known this for a while, it's been too early to say anything to anyone else. I've been struggling to keep it a secret and not blurt it out in a tic at some inopportune moment. Laura's started to tell other people now though, and tonight she told Emma.

I'm relieved the risk of Tourettes stealing Laura's thunder has passed, and I'm so excited about her news. The immediate result was that I kept ticcing, 'Emma's pregnant' and 'I'm pregnant' while we were out.

HEADS UP

I've re-entered a head-banging phase. Not the music-related throwing-your-hair-about type but the fist-to-head variety. This has happened intermittently before but it's become pretty regular over the last couple of days. This head-banging doesn't stop even if I'm holding something in my hands. Already today I've hit my forehead with: a phone, a carton of apple juice, a set of keys, a toilet roll dispenser and a strawberry.

I BREAK

On Thursday while I was working on my laptop I ticced and head-butted the top of the screen. The bridge of my nose hit the thin metal edge which was incredibly painful. I felt a massive lump come up almost immediately, but thankfully Leftwing Idiot was equally quick at getting some frozen peas to help ease the swelling and make me look less like an extra from Star Trek.

But when I woke up this morning the swelling and bruising

looked much more dramatic than it had yesterday. I'd got double black eyes again and one eyelid was so swollen it wasn't opening properly. I panicked and called Fat Sister, who's a doctor and didn't answer straightaway because she was at work. By the time she called back I'd got over the shock of seeing my bashed-up looking face and was feeling less worried. Nevertheless, Fat Sister wanted me to get a doctor to have a look at it. I've ignored her advice before and regretted it, so I made my way to the nearest Minor Injuries Unit.

I got stunning service, just as I did at my local hospital when I twisted my ankle a while back. The outcome is that it's quite likely I've broken my nose but they're not too worried about it. There's not much they can do about a broken nose it seems, but they've made a clinic appointment for me in a couple of weeks in case there are any persistent problems once the swelling's gone down.

While I can wholeheartedly recommend the NHS's outstanding service, I really need to try and stay out of A&E.

And while I can wholeheartedly recommend shiny metal laptops, I really need to avoid head-butting mine.

DLA

A letter arrived this morning to say I've been awarded Disability Living Allowance. DLA is a benefit that helps cover the additional costs of having a disability. I'll get a backdated payment from when I applied, and I've worked out that this pretty much matches what I've spent since then on things to limit the impact of the tics, like gloves and plastic cutlery.

But it doesn't come close to what I've spent on travel, on replacing things I've broken or on my friends' expenses' when they've helped me do something I couldn't do on my own.

DLA will mean that I can continue to get the things I need to keep me safe and improve the quality of my life. That's if the government don't get there first.

DREAMS INTERRUPTED

My tics can make it hard for me to settle down and get to sleep, but usually I only wake up a couple of times during the night. Every now and again, though, I'll wake up over and over again and that's what happened last night. I'm not sure if it's the ticcing that wakes me, or if I tic just as I wake up. Either way, being wrenched from sleep, time after time, squealing, shouting or jerking, is quite a shock and really frustrating. Last night, by the time I'd woken for the twentieth time, I felt pretty desperate.

At least it's the weekend, which should give me plenty of time to catch up on sleep.

MAY

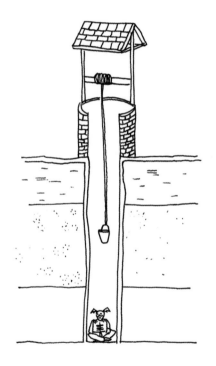

HEIP, I'M STUCK DOWN A WELL.

AMAZING

A new tic emerged tonight and it's literally 'Amazing!'

'Cream crackers are amazing!'
'Crime is amazing!'
'Ladders are amazing!'
'Bribery is amazing!'
'*I'm* amazing!'

THERE'S SOMEBODY AT THE DOOR

This morning I was enjoying a relaxing start to the day when the doorbell rang.

RING 1

It was a courier with a letter for Fat Sister. He looked flustered and awkward as I jerked about in the doorway. I signed for the letter and he went on his way.

Moments later the doorbell went again.

RING 2

This time it was a political campaigner with a clipboard, canvassing for a local election. I listened attentively while shouting 'Yay, sheepdogs!' He didn't try to count on my vote for long.

I hadn't even sat down when it rang again.

RING 3

It was two people from a local church, offering me individual bible study sessions. They looked very relieved when I didn't take them up on their offer.

Unsolicited visits are unusual at the lair, but I suspect they're more of a surprise for the people ringing the bell. There can't be women shouting about biscuits behind many doors.

The doorbell rang again.

RING 4

This time I was greeted warmly by our regular postman. He knows exactly what to expect and was smiling and friendly as he handed me a parcel.

SUPPORTED

I've already mentioned the amazing treatment I've been having recently at my local hospital. Since my tic-related ankle injury I've had help from several different departments there, and the care they've given has been fantastic.

This morning I went for an orthotics appointment, arranged by my physiotherapist. The orthotics team make braces and splints for pretty much any part of the body, and they're going to provide me with supports to help stabilise my walking.

The orthotist was brilliant. He listened attentively as I described the impact of tics on my mobility and asked me what I thought would help. He's ordered some supports for my ankles and some discreet padding for my knees. The plan is to try these less intrusive options first, and if they don't work effectively, we can try a more comprehensive leg brace.

We also discussed the possibility of using a compression suit. These are used by people with a range of conditions, particularly children with autism or cerebral palsy. The orthotist said you need to take loads of measurements to make them, which isn't always easy, and although he's used to dealing with wriggly kids, he thought he'd need a strong cup of coffee before trying to measure me.

SURPRISE

It's two weeks until King Russell's birthday.

I bought his present – an expensive but brilliant Star Wars cap – about two months ago. He loves Star Wars and has lots of clothing featuring characters from the films. A particular favourite of his is a Storm Trooper t-shirt he wears all the time. Every time he's worn it recently I've ticced: 'I've bought you a ...' Up until now I've been able to stop myself saying anything more. Today I completed the sentence with '... hat.'

I'm not sure how I'm going to maintain the surprise until his birthday. Fortunately I also ticced: 'I've bought you a helicopter.' 'I've bought you a standing ovation for Christmas.' And 'I've bought you an ovarian cyst.'

Hopefully he'll have no idea which one's the real gift.

TIME FOR TODDLERS

I hung out with Owain, the Tourettes-loving toddler, again this evening. I was saying 'Bye, bye' a lot but he soon got used to the idea that I wasn't going anywhere.

He was absolutely fascinated by my boxing gloves and enjoyed trying them on. Unfortunately, he's also started repeating a tic that might not go down brilliantly at nursery: 'Baby dogging.'

Hopefully his mum will understand.

TAKING THE BISCUIT

(The words in grey are the actual tics that came out while I was trying to write – please concentrate on the black text.)

Biscuit, biscuit, biscuit I'm going biscuit to do I'm a biscuit tonight's entry biscuit slightly differently. I love biscuits Normally biscuits writing is the only time my biscuits love biscuits tics don't get in the way biscuit of what I'm trying to say biscuit, biscuit because biscuit I don't include them. But biscuit tonight my entry biscuit, biscuit is about my frustration with biscuits so I'm a biscuit, biscuit, biscuit I'm writing down every time I tic biscuit biscuit-related tics.

This evening bisscuuiiit I was working on something with biscuit I'm a biscuit Leftwing Idiot biscuuuittts and because I was exhausted and frustrated, I was struggling to biscuit concentrate. Biscuit, biscuit, biscuit, biscuit I fought to get my thoughts clear in my mind and explain the points I wanted biscuit to make I love biscuits but this was made extremely difficult by my tics. Hands up if you love biscuits. Squares love biscuits.

In the end Leftwing Idiot called a halt to what we were biscuit doing biscuit and said we were biscuit both too worn out to carry on. Biscuit, biscuit I started to cry, he gave me a hug biscuit and like all good hugs when you're upset, this made me cry more.

Biscuit I felt overwhelmingly frustrated and as I sobbed I continued to shout 'biscuit' busy biscuit. All I wanted was to stop saying biscuit – but I couldn't. What I did say biscuuuuitsss, biscies was: 'Don't say biscuits. Biscuits,' followed by, 'If you say biscuit one more time I'm going to kill you. Biscuit.' I love biscuits.

For the record, I'm totally indifferent to biscuits.

'KICK YOUR LOVE LIFE IN THE BACKSIDE'

I've had a busy day travelling across the city to meet up with various friends. I had dinner by the river and went to my friends' post-wedding party. It's been an enjoyable day shared with lots of different people.

For a good part of it I was with Leftwing Idiot. While we were walking along the river he started to rib me about fancying someone or other. As the conversation went on I told him that I find myself feeling lonely.

This clearly stayed on his mind because he came back to it again later. I explained that although I'm generally happy on my own, I sometimes miss having a romantic interest.

Although I don't believe I'm single because I have Tourettes, I do think a man might need considerable vision to find a woman who shouts 'biscuit' and thumps herself a lot sexy.

I know feeling lonely is a common experience. For lots of people, including me, it isn't something that's constant or crushing, but I know there are many others for whom it's a much bigger problem.

Perhaps I'm just Bridget Jones with swearing and I'll have a Hollywood ending to look forward to. Perhaps I won't. Either way, I'm lucky to have the friends I've got.

SQUAWKING IN THE POND

This afternoon I went swimming with Harry – she's a friend of ours who lives nearby with her boyfriend Ollie.

'Ollie has hair.'
'Ollie has a little bear.'
'Ollie go to bed.'

It's been baking hot in London so we went straight to Hampstead Ponds, to swim with the ducks, geese and moorhens. The water was ink black and freezing. I was terrified because I couldn't touch the bottom. Concentrating on making rhythmic, controlled movements supported by the water helps me to feel more in control of my body so I love swimming.

While we were holding onto a buoyancy aid having a rest, an elderly woman swam up to us and said, 'I wouldn't want to be your neighbour – you're so noisy I could hear you from the other side of the water.' I said, 'Sorry if I was disturbing you,' and explained I couldn't control the noises or movements I was making. She didn't appear to understand, despite me trying to describe it in a number of different ways.

She swam around us a few times looking sceptical. After several minutes of circling she looked at me directly and said, 'Tourettes Syndrome.' I confirmed that she was correct.

A BITE FOR BREAKFAST

When I was younger I had a tic that made me bite my sister. This would often happen when we were sitting next to each other at meal times. I haven't done this for years but this morning I was standing behind her in the kitchen when I ticced, 'I'm not going to bite you!'

Without turning round she said, 'Don't think I didn't hear your teeth snapping.'

She was right – I'd gone for her arm but caught myself just in time.

I've had biting tics on and off since I was a child. A couple of months ago I started biting my hands and arms a lot which was obviously painful for me but also distressing for other people. To help with this I used a technique I learnt during Habit Reversal Therapy. Each time I went to take a bite I made myself do an opposing movement with my arm and my mouth. This meant putting my hand behind my back and doing a gentle kiss with my lips. Things quickly improved and I became much more aware of the tic. Soon I was managing to catch myself before I sank my teeth in.

Sadly, this technique didn't work quickly enough to save Leftwing Idiot's phone. It hasn't worked properly since I bit it.

PINEAPPLES OR ARMS?

PART ONE

There are two pineapples in the kitchen left over from a party last week. They're on the turn and need to be eaten soon.

I really fancy pineapple for breakfast this morning but no one's around to help me cut them up. I can't do it safely myself at the moment because my arm tics mean I can't control the knife. The pineapples are too tough for plastic cutlery so I'd need to use a metal blade.

Do I risk it with the kitchen knife or let the pineapples go to waste?

PART TWO

I shared my fruity dilemma with Harry in the end and she stopped by the lair and sliced them up for me. We spent the rest of the afternoon together in the park eating delicious pineapple chunks.

INDEPENDENCE DAY

I've already described what a lifeline the Disability Living Allowance is proving to be. But I haven't yet mentioned Access to Work. This is a scheme that helps disabled people in employment by funding the specialised support or equipment they might need to do their jobs more effectively.

I applied for Access to Work a while back and today, for the first time, I was joined at work by Leftwing Idiot, who's taken on the task of being my new support worker. He'll be helping me a couple of times a week by coming to meetings and events with me and taking notes or typing whenever necessary. We've not worked together for a long time but I'm glad I've been able to choose the person I want to support me rather than having to get used to someone new. My arm tics are making it increasingly difficult for me to do these tasks myself, and this help will mean I'll be able to work just as quickly as someone without Tourettes.

In addition, Access to Work has agreed to fund my transport to and from work. My tics have made using public transport increasingly difficult – I often need to get off one bus and onto another several times per journey because of other people's adverse reactions. This can make even simple journeys long, stressful and expensive. I clearly need a reliable way of getting to work, and the cabs they've agreed to fund should make a big difference.

In the past I've felt uncomfortable about the idea of getting extra help and I've worried about what other people would think about it. But I've realised there's no point struggling just for the sake of it, if help is available.

I read an article by Laurence Clark on the BBC Ouch website that mirrors how I feel: 'Today I guess I've realised that living independently has nothing to do with doing everything ourselves without help, or living in isolation. It's about us controlling our own lifestyles by making choices, taking decisions and managing our own support, as non-disabled people do every day.'

CRACKING THE SAFE

By my desk at work there's a safe. I don't have to use it very often, but I check it's locked many times a day. I do this out of habit. I've always been slightly obsessive about checking things, and it's not as bad as it was when I was younger. Then, I used to check things over and over again. For example, my family got used to hearing the test beep of the smoke alarm every night.

This obsessive behaviour didn't stop at checking electrical equipment. Each time my Gran taught me a new prayer at bedtime I added it to a long list of others I felt I had to say before I could go to sleep. In the end there were five or six I had to get through every night.

As I got older these rituals became less of a problem and I was able to reason my way out of them. I still allow myself to do these sorts of things a bit though, particularly when they're harmless, like checking the safe or counting things I can see. The back window at Leftwing Idiot's flat looks out over the gardens and houses beyond. I love the view from this window and if I'm there with a moment to spare I start to count. At night it's the lit windows in the houses and on a summer's day it's the pears on a nearby tree. The big difference between now and when I was a child is that now I can make myself stop if I need to.

I don't have Obsessive Compulsive Disorder (OCD), though it's quite a common condition amongst people with Tourettes. For people with OCD, repetitive thoughts and actions are a much bigger problem and can be debilitating, or even paralysing. For me, obsessive tendencies can sometimes have a positive value. For example, they can help me focus on completing big work tasks efficiently.

Even though my obsessive behaviour doesn't impact on my life very much any more, I've decided to have a zero tolerance policy from now on. So today I didn't check the safe. I went to do it, but caught myself in time. Leftwing Idiot tested my resolve. As we left to go home he asked, 'Don't you want to check the safe?' I told him I didn't want to because I knew it was locked. 'Are you sure? It might be open.' I laughed and said, 'No, it's fine.'

KINDNESS IN A CAB

When I got in a cab to come home this evening, the driver was startled by the noise I was making and looked quite scared. I explained about Tourettes and a little later he said, 'I don't care if you're offended, but I've got to say I've never met anyone like you before.' We chatted about Tourettes, and about how he was finding the switch from driving a bus to driving a cab. He was a lovely guy and shortly before I got out he said, 'You're good, don't let anyone tell you any different.'

TOURETTES AND YOU KNOW IT

The Tourettes language-generating machine swung into frenzied action this evening to the tune of 'If you're happy and you know it.' The following tics all arrived in the first half hour and I repeated them at full blast for several hours more:

'Norma Major's in your mouth, take a bite.'
'There's a ferret in your soul, cut it out.'
'Derren Brown's in the room, shut your mind.'
'There's a dog in your wallet, wash your hands.'
'Eamonn Holmes's in your mum, kick him out.'
'There's a squirrel in your pants, have a bath.'
'There's a man in your bed, hose him down.'

I'm happy and I know it but I'm not so sure about my neighbours.

NIGHT

I'm absolutely exhausted because I haven't slept properly for weeks and the last few days have been particularly difficult and frustrating. I keep waking myself up thrashing about and shouting.

Getting to sleep's been a problem for ages but my tics haven't been repeatedly waking me up throughout the night in the way they are at the moment. My lack of sleep's been affecting how well I can function during the day, so tonight I'm going to try a new medication prescribed by my doctor. It's called Melatonin and I'm hoping it helps because the current situation isn't sustainable.

STUCK

I went to the pub this evening with Harry, Ollie, Fat Sister and King Russell. I didn't stay long though because I was wriggling about all over the place. The pub's only five minutes from the lair so I thought I'd be able to make it back on my own.

In fact it took me twenty-five minutes, and at one point it felt like I wasn't going to make it. The problem is my squatting-down tic – it's been around for a while but recently it's become more frequent. It feels like being pulled suddenly to the ground and it's making getting about even trickier than usual.

I'M APPALLING! I'M AMAZING!

A while ago I mentioned I'd started ticing 'I'm amazing!' That's now been joined by 'I'm appalling!'

I made myself laugh as I struggled up the stairs to the lair tonight, calling each one out in turn.

IS IT OK?

It's OK to laugh at the woman shouting as she goes up the escalator at the station because you're with your mates and you're sharing a funny moment.

It's OK to sit in your car and laugh at the girl walking strangely as she crosses the road, because you're bored and you're never going to see her again.

It's OK to whisper comments about the jerky woman because she probably can't hear or understand what you're saying.

It's OK to film on your phone someone behaving weirdly because your mates will find it funny later and you want them to like you.

It's OK to sit quietly and not do anything when fifteen teenagers laugh at someone with a disability, because you're scared.

It's OK to stay sitting down in the priority seat when someone who can't stand properly gets on the bus, because they're swearing and don't deserve your help.

If you think like this you're not alone. Your look, laugh or comment joins millions of others up and down the country.

But there was one man today whose reaction was different.

It really is OK that you asked me if I had Tourettes. Chatting to you was interesting and made both our journeys more enjoyable, and I was happy to answer your questions.

Thanks for your empathy.

ALL QUIET AT THE LAIR

Tonight the lair seems massive and echoey. The piles of stuff that have been a feature for the last month have all gone. Fat Sister and King Russell moved out yesterday in preparation for married life.

Fat Sister, King Russell and I have lived together at the lair for four years, and during that time my tics have intensified considerably. I'm worried I might have underestimated how much support they give me. Fortunately they haven't moved far.

Before they left to spend the first night in their new home they gave me a list of instructions:

1) Don't lock the bathroom door
2) Wear shoes if you use the kettle (so it hurts less if you pour boiling water over your feet)
3) Don't try to go up or down stairs without help
4) The oven is not your friend – don't use it
5) Always keep your phone to hand and call us if you need to

So now I'm living on my own. It feels strange and it's making me sad and tearful. I don't want to live by myself for long, and I'm planning to get new flatmates soon. But that won't be here because I've decided to move out and put the lair up for sale.

At the moment I have to negotiate four flights of stairs to get home and there are more once I'm inside. This is far from ideal because my tics make it hard for me to move around safely on my own. On balance it seems sensible to look for somewhere that's easier to manage.

JUNE

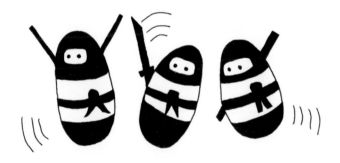

NINJAS WOBBLE BUT THEY DON'T FALL DOWN.

WHAT HAPPENS IF YOU SWEAR IN BARNSLEY?

Simple. You risk getting an on-the-spot fine of £80.

During June, Barnsley police are having a crackdown on swearing in public. I'm one of the 10% of people with Tourettes who swear involuntarily, so I took a particular interest in this story.

Several of my friends with Tourettes joked that we should go to Barnsley for our next outing.

SELF-SHOCKED

While a lot of my tics are random and funny, occasionally they come across as just rude or mean. It doesn't happen very often but sometimes I'll suddenly say something like, 'Bitch', 'Fuck you' or 'Wanker', and these are much closer to the stereotype of Tourettes than the majority of my tics.

It shocks me when this happens and I worry people might think it's directed at them, even if they know I have Tourettes. Last week I was staying at my mum's and having just said goodnight to her I said, 'Piss off, bitch.' I don't know if she heard me or not – she didn't react – but I felt I had to go and say goodnight to her again to make sure everything was all right.

MAKING HIS PARENTS PROUD

My leg tics mean I'm walking in ways that look increasingly unusual and dramatic. I have much less control than I used to and frequently find myself dropping to the floor. Surprisingly, very few people who see this ask if I'm OK. I suspect this is either because I don't look fazed by it or because the screeching noises and jerky movements I'm making at the same time scare people off.

None of this put off a boy in the supermarket this afternoon though. He was about eleven and out shopping with his family, although they weren't there when I walked erratically past and dropped down in the aisle near him. He didn't think twice about coming to help me. I was in a rush, so I thanked him quickly, but didn't mention why I'd dropped down in any detail.

I regretted this, and while I was waiting outside for a cab I saw him leave with his parents. I approached them and told them how kind he'd been. It also gave me an opportunity to thank him properly and explain why I'd fallen. His mum and dad were clearly pleased and I was glad I'd taken the time to show my appreciation of the spontaneous care he'd shown me.

MINISTRY OF SILLY WALKS

A couple of days ago I got a copy of a letter to my GP from my neurologist. In the letter he describes how my tics are affecting the way I walk. He said it looked like 'The Ministry of Silly Walks'.

I'm used to people who are unfamiliar with Tourettes making thoughtless remarks, but I didn't expect to get a comment like this from my own neurologist. After reading the letter I've started feeling much more self-conscious about the way I walk.

I'm fairly certain that a doctor wouldn't describe a wheelchair user as looking like Andy from 'Little Britain', or someone with a visual impairment being like Mr Magoo.

DOUBLE TALK

It's a week until Fat Sister and King Russell's wedding and tonight I finished writing my speech. I'm Maid of Honour and although it's not standard for the chief bridesmaid to speak, Fat Sister wants at least one speech from a woman.

However carefully honed my words are on the page, only half of what I say will have been written down. The other, ticced, half is an unknown quantity and will be as much a surprise to me as to everybody else.

I'd put money on there being some 'biscuits' in there though.

STUCK TO THE FLOOR

The dropping-to-the-floor tic is happening more frequently and I'm finding it much harder to get around. This has left me feeling stranded and frustrated.

However tricky new tics are, once I get used to them they become easier to manage and I find ways of living with them. I'm taking practical steps to limit the risks from this tic by sleeping downstairs and wearing kneepads. The kneepads don't just protect me – they also protect my clothes. I'm wearing them over my jeans because I've destroyed two pairs this week already.

THE REAL ROYAL WEDDING

The real royal wedding started early with a cup of tea at Fat Sister's new flat. We had a few calm minutes together before her wedding day began in earnest.

DRESSES

As a doctor, Fat Sister's great at making quick decisions, but if she's given more time she's the most indecisive person I know. Her wedding dress has been an ongoing issue for several months now. She'd whittled it down to two white dresses this morning but hadn't made a choice by the time I'd left. I had to wait until she turned up at the registry office to find out which one she'd gone for.

She wasn't the only one wearing white – her bridesmaids were too. White isn't a Tourettes-friendly colour, but I managed to keep my outfit clean all day except for one green streak down the back from where I'd suddenly dropped down and sat on a plant pot.

THE CEREMONY

The entrance music started and Fat Sister walked in with my dad.

TH: Here comes the sheep.

Registrar: If any person knows of any lawful impediment to this marriage they should declare it now.

TH: Don't worry, they're not siblings!

Registrar: Do you Fat Sister take King Russell to be your lawfully wedded husband?

Fat Sister: I do.

TH: Including the eyebrows?

Fat Sister told me later that the registrar, who was brilliant, had wiped away a tear of laughter at this point.

THE SPEECH

Hello and good afternoon, biscuit, for anyone who doesn't know me, I'm a biscuit, I'm Fat Sister's sister. If you don't know me, biscuit, biscuit, this speech will make a lot more sense, biscuit, if you also know I have, biscuits, Tourettes.

Some of this speech is planned and some of it, keys, will be a surprise to all, biscuits, of us including me. It is likely to contain many biscuits and a number of, biscuit, inaccuracies.

For the record: they're not siblings. King Russell, biscuit, didn't break the shower. He's not able to read minds, biscuit, hasn't to the best of my knowledge, biscuit, fallen out of a wormhole, or taken a bullet for my mum. Biscuit. He has however been engaged to my sister, keys, fuck, fuck, biscuit, Happy Christmas, biscuit.

It's evident to all who meet them, biscuit, they have a solid, loving, balanced relationship and should be together always.

Biscuit. A relationship which started exactly, biscuit, 42 years ago, biscuit, biscuit, that's not strictly true, exactly eleven years ago. Biscuit. A quick shout out to Lee who was there at the beginning on 17th June 2000, biscuit.

One of Fat Sister's friends, biscuit, determined to find her a boyfriend, fuck, biscuit, biscuit, had organised a party for prospective suitors. King Russell arrived first. Biscuit, biscuit, biscuit.

It's been a privilege, biscuit, to see each of them, biscuit, and their relationship, biscuit, flourish, biscuits, biscuit, develop and, biscuit, strengthen. Fuck. Having lived with them, biscuit, biscuit, I've seen, biscuit, I've seen them have sex! Just remember the inaccuracies bit. Keys, keys, I've got to find my place again now.

Having lived with them, biscuit, I've seen, biscuit, biscuit, day in day out, how caring, thoughtful and perfectly matched they are, biscuit, biscuit, biscuit. It also means I know:

Never to ask King Russell to change the position of his desk, biscuit, biscuit.

That if Fat Sister, biscuit, discovers a hissing gas leak, Transco will be her fourth call, eeeek, ahhh, biscuit, biscuit.

That, biscuit, there's, biscuit, no alarm, biscuit, on earth that can wake King Russell up.

That Fat Sister, biscuit, biscuit, ahhhh, is a skilful first aider, especially when drunk.

That they have many shared loves: Come Dine With Me, biscuit, mini Babybels, Buffy the Vampire Slayer, biscuit, sleeping, biscuit.

Recently, biscuit, Fat Sister, biscuit, told me she'd been at a party with King Russell about a year, biscuit, after they'd first started dating. Fuck, biscuit, biscuit. She'd turned to him and drunkenly said, biscuit, 'I think we'll still be doing this together in ten years time.' Today proves she was right. Biscuit, biscuit.

I knew King Russell was serious about Fat Sister when he bought her an iPod for Christmas. Most of you will be aware how much he hates Apple, but he knew it would make her squeal with glee. Hi, boof, biscuit, boof, hoof, hoof. King Russell, biscuit, you are, biscuit, thoughtful, calm and patient in everything you do, or in Fat Sister's words, 'You're awesome.' Biscuit, biscuit, biscuit, biscuit, biscuit.

Anyone, biscuit, who's heard Fat Sister, biscuit, discuss her role in King Russell's zombie plan will know, biscuit, she's clearly committed to their relationship, fuck.

Fat Sister, you are generous, compassionate and kind, biscuit. You have always had a mind of your own, biscuit, and an innate sense of good and what's right, biscuit. Your humour, biscuit, and spirit of, biscuits, adventure make you a great, biscuit, sister, biscuit, friend, biscuit, and potential zombie-fighting partner. Fuck off.

Biscuit, on behalf of all your bridesmaids, ahh, biscuit, I would like to say, Fat Sister you look beautiful, and to King Russell we're really pleased we're not dressed as Orks.

It's been an amazing day, keys, and we're proud to have been part of this landmark in your, biscuit, lives together. Biscuit, biscuit. Today is a celebration of all you've achieved and shared so far, biscuit, as well as all that is to come, biscuit. Wishing you many more years of love and happiness together. Fuck, fuck, biscuit.

To Fat Sister and King Russell.

Inevitably, my tics interrupted all the other speeches too. I told my dad not to make jokes, and ticced the punch lines to the best man's anecdotes.

It's been a perfect day.

'WHO'S YOUR FAVOURITE CARER -- ANGEL GABRIEL OR JOHN LEWIS?'

It's National Carers Week and while I'm writing this, Poppy's in the other room cooking up a storm. She's making dinner for tonight and also stuff to freeze which I can eat in the next few days. The food I'm able to prepare safely by myself is limited because it's dangerous for me to use anything sharper than a plastic knife. Pouring, carrying and stirring can be messy too if you add uncontrollable arm tics, and getting ingredients in the first place is tricky because my leg tics have a big impact on my mobility. Leftwing Idiot did some shopping for me earlier and I now have cupboards full of food.

Poppy, Leftwing Idiot, Fat Sister and King Russell will all be away from tomorrow and they're the people I rely on the most. It hadn't dawned on me until just now, but their thoughtfulness means I'll have all the key stuff I need while I'm on my own.

I've always felt uncomfortable with the term 'carer' and tend to use 'personal assistant' or 'support worker'. But none of these words adequately describes the kindness and consideration I'm shown every day by my friends.

Recent research estimates unpaid carers save the UK £119 billion a year. The Carers UK website features a care calculator that allows people to see the estimated value of the care they provide. I used it to see how much the care I receive would cost. The total was £59,130 per year. Rather than looking after this incredibly valuable national resource, the Government's sweeping spending cuts are putting carers under ever-increasing strain.

I don't always find it easy to accept the care I'm given, and I sometimes get upset when other people draw attention to it. I worry about the responsibility helping me places on my friends and I get frustrated by all the things that having Tourettes makes difficult.

But I don't feel worried or upset today – I just feel incredibly touched by the thoughtfulness my friends have shown me. I'm also very excited by the pea and mint risotto, pasta sauce and vegetable stew just going into the freezer.

FLOORED

I've written about how frequently I'm now dropping to the floor, and how this is making getting about difficult. Most tics are rapid movements, but what's unusual about this one is that I'm finding it difficult to get out of it independently. This tic seems to involve a very quick movement to start with, sometimes followed by a more sustained movement that twists my body onto the ground.

Tonight, at the lair on my own, I dropped down and ended up on the floor making a series of rapidly repeating movements that meant I was wiggling about all over the place and couldn't get up safely. I used the exercises I'd learnt in Habit Reversal Therapy to try and re-establish control but it still took well over ten minutes for me to get to my feet.

TAKING THE STRAIN

Leftwing Idiot got back from his trip this evening and I went for some food with him, Poppy and our friend Belle, who's come to stay at the lair for a few days.

It's been boiling, but I couldn't move anywhere without wearing thick kneepads and clinging sweatily to my friends. Each time I dropped down, they caught my weight and I could hear them let out a breath from the exertion.

As Leftwing Idiot and I struggled up the stairs to the lair he said, 'It's not getting any better, is it?' I agreed. It's a fair observation. I felt a wave of desperation. These tics might go on for days, weeks, months or even years. They'll either get better, or worse, or I'll get used to them. But the worry that's always at the back of my mind is that new tics can turn up unannounced at any time and completely disrupt my life and routines.

'ARE YOU A SPASTIC?'

It's been baking hot in London, and along with everybody else I've been out enjoying the sunshine. It seems like the better the weather the more unusual the questions from strangers become.

Man at bus stop: Are you a spastic?
TH: No, I don't have cerebral palsy. I have Tourettes.

Man in shop: Shouldn't you be in hospital?
TH: No, I'm not ill.

Man on bus: Why don't you just shut up?

I'm generally happy when people ask me questions about my tics. Today's questions were less welcome but they didn't make my blood boil, the sun was doing that for me.

'NINJAS WOBBLE BUT THEY DON'T FALL DOWN'

Leftwing Idiot came round to the lair and Belle cooked an amazing dinner. Later, I went upstairs with Leftwing Idiot to fetch something. I've hardly been upstairs for weeks, and he asked, 'While we're up here is there anything else you need?' I sat on the bed thinking about what to take downstairs while I had the opportunity.

We started to talk about the difficulties I'm having getting around and how I'm approaching them. He told me how frustrated he feels that I'm not prioritising the things that would help me deal with these difficulties, like getting on with selling the lair, or sorting out a regular food delivery.

I cried, but it was more out of exasperation than sadness. We went back downstairs, had a bit of chocolate and chatted to Belle.

As I write this I realise on a positive note that I didn't over-react. Although having Tourettes is basically constant, different aspects of it shift unpredictably and have more or less impact on my life.

WHOSE LEARNING DISABILITY?

I called the local social care team earlier to check they'd received the form I'd sent them describing the difficulties I'm experiencing at the moment. The friendly woman I spoke to confirmed they'd got it but said they'd be passing it on to the learning disability team.

TH: Why?
Social Worker: Because we don't deal with Tourettes.
TH: But I don't have a learning disability.
Social Worker: My manager said we have to pass it on to the learning disability team.
TH: But I really *don't* have a learning disability. My difficulties are mainly to do with mobility.
Social Worker: Hang on – let me talk to my manager.
Social Work Manager: Hello?
TH: Hi. Your colleague told me you've received my self-assessment but are planning to pass it to the learning disability team. I'm confused because I don't have a learning disability.
Social Work Manager: I know Tourettes isn't technically a learning disability, but they deal with conditions like Aspergers. We only deal with physical disabilities.
TH: I have a neurological condition and my involuntary movements are my biggest problem. They're physically disabling and seriously affect my independence. Socially and intellectually I'm fine, I just can't get up and down stairs.
Social Work Manager: The learning disability team will be able to help you better. They might be able to help you manage your tics.

TH: How? I have all the medical care I need and they're not going to be able to do anything a neurologist can't. I need practical help and support.

Social Work Manager: We provide aids and equipment and stuff. We won't really be able to help you.

TH: So you don't provide people with support workers?

Social Work Manager: Well, we do, but normally for things like help around the home or with going shopping if someone can't walk easily.

TH: That's what I need. I'm living in unsuitable accommodation. I have a job I love and some support at work, but my mobility's deteriorated and I'm dependent on friends for help. I'm really not managing on a practical level. I understand there's not going to be a dedicated Tourettes team, but I would've thought the best way to assess me would be to look at the nature of the problems I'm experiencing. At the moment mine are mainly linked to my mobility.

Social Work Manager: I take your point and I'll discuss it with the other managers here and the manager of the learning disability team, and get back to you.

TH: Thank you.

Which team finally provides the help isn't important if the support I need is provided, but I've worked in social services and know the learning disability team isn't going to accept my case because I won't meet their eligibility criteria. I'll have to wait and see.

CHILD CARE

Today I've had three lovely interactions with children being thoughtful, caring and considerate towards me.

At work I talked to a seven-year-old girl whom I'd not met before. While we were saying hello and introducing ourselves I explained about having Tourettes. She was clearly interested.

Girl: You must be really special. I wish I were you and said 'biscuit', and 'keys'.

TH: You're the first person that's ever said that.

(She smiled)

Girl: I like how you move, but I know it's hard too.

After work a friend of mine and her teenage son who has Down Syndrome gave me a lift back to the lair. When we arrived her son insisted she should help me up the stairs, and he wouldn't get back in the car until I'd waved at him from the balcony to show I was safe.

Later, as I was coming back from the shops, some of the local children came and had a chat. They're always thoughtful and tonight we talked about me dropping to the floor and my kneepads. The girl who lives below me said, 'I think maybe you should live on the ground floor.' I agreed, and all eight of them came up the stairs with me to make sure I was all right.

JULY

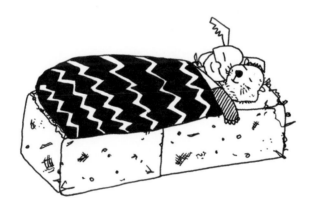

I LOVE YOU MR OTTER.

HAPPY CHRISTMAS

'Calm down Christmas time.'
  'Do you think I'm a Christmas tree?'
  'God hates Christmas.'
  'Runner, runner, runner, runner, Christmas bean.'

… it's July.

SWEARING WITH FATHER

I was chatting with my dad on the phone today. He's obviously used to our conversations being peppered with tics, including lots of swearing which he never seems to mind. Today's conversation was no exception, until halfway through I described something as being 'Fucking awful'. He knew this wasn't a tic and told me to mind my language. I laughed.

Anyone who thinks having Tourettes means you can get away with swearing hasn't met my dad.

THE EARTH MOVED

I've spent the day building a sandpit at one of the projects I work at. This involved digging a big hole and then filling it with rubble, using a JCB.

The therapeutic benefits of JCB driving might not be immediately apparent, but I found it surprisingly calming. There are lots of different things to push and turn but the JCB responded quite slowly so when I ticced it didn't mess things up or get dangerous.

My colleague, who was working with me, even commented that my digging was 'Very controlled', and that isn't something I hear said about me often!

It was loads of fun and it's good to know that although I might not be able to cut up a pineapple I can dig a very big hole.

STROPPY

It's been a bad day, not specifically because of Tourettes but just one of those days that doesn't feel like it's going right. Because I felt moody and unsettled I was particularly unpleasant to Leftwing Idiot, and this led to a row.

Our argument, like others we've had, was complicated by my need for help with my tics. I felt furious, but at the same time I needed him to hold my hands to stop me thumping myself. My mood improved later in the day when we sat in the park and made our peace.

Sometimes physical dependence like this makes it hard to establish the distance and perspective necessary for resolving a disagreement. Occasionally though it's absolutely necessary for letting me *have* an argument.

A while ago King Russell held my hands to stop me scratching my face during a heated discussion I was having with Fat Sister. His help meant I could have a good shout at his wife without anyone getting injured.

MIDNIGHT FEAST WITH THE POLICE

Leftwing Idiot and I were out all day. On the way home we headed to our local kebab shop to get something to eat. There was a police car outside and we could see two officers ordering dinner at the counter. Leftwing Idiot took a deep breath as he opened the door and said, 'This is going to be interesting.'

Police always make my tics worse.

I ordered our food and we sat down to wait. It only took a minute for my tics to catch their attention. The cops looked shocked and stared at me disapprovingly. This wasn't much of a surprise. In addition to my normal repertoire of 'biscuits' 'keys' and 'fuck', their presence had triggered a whole farmyard full of pig noises that I was trying desperately to stifle.

After ten long uncomfortable minutes they left with their food. I'd like to have heard what they said on their way back to the car.

THE LONG AND SHORT WALK OF IT

I suddenly realised this afternoon that I needed to go to the bank, but, although it's only five minutes away, the prospect of walking there alone filled me with dread. It's not a day when I have support at work so I had to go by myself, and inevitably I kept dropping to the ground. Unusually, I was offered some help from passers-by today – one man even asked me if I'd like a lift on his bike. I got there and back successfully in the end, but it was tricky.

I've always enjoyed walking – it's been my favourite way of getting around since I learned how to do it. As a teenager I enjoyed going on long walks by myself, and in my mind I still do.

Now, I have to steel myself to walk anywhere. I know I'll keep crashing to the ground but I'm never sure when, and each time it happens it's a shock. But though the practical difficulties are certainly challenging, what I miss most is the peace, and time to think, that I used to get from this simple activity.

THE MR OTTER AFFAIR

Poppy and Leftwing Idiot came over earlier to pick something up from the lair.

Poppy: What are you going to do this afternoon?
TH: Some drawing, read the paper, have sex with an otter.
Leftwing Idiot: OK. When's *that* happening?
TH: I'm going to wake him up.
Leftwing Idiot: Is Mr Otter upstairs now?
TH: Cuddle Mr Otter.

My friends and my tics carried on talking about my otter lover all day.

I love you Mr Otter.

DISABILITY AWARENESS TRAINING

I've been at a disability awareness training course all day. Because I hadn't received a letter asking if I needed any additional support, when I arrived I explained to the trainer that I had Tourettes. 'Well, if I can't handle that I shouldn't be doing this job,' she said.

After she'd introduced herself, she asked each of us to say a bit about ourselves. The first woman who spoke gave her name and told us where she worked. Then she gestured at me and said, 'I assume that lady has Tourettes, and I just need to say that I might leave the room if it gets too much.'

The trainer asked me how I felt about this, and I said it was fine, but addressing the woman I said, 'You know I can't control the noises or movements I make don't you?' She said she did, and the introductions continued round the table.

While I always encourage people to be open with me, the woman's comment left me feeling uncomfortable. Whenever I introduce myself I always introduce Tourettes too, on my own terms. I felt like my control over that had been undermined.

The rest of the session was interesting and the trainer encouraged me to share my experiences at relevant points. During a break she asked if I would consider delivering similar training with her in the future. I told her I'd think about it.

In reality, every day involves me doing disability awareness training of some kind, whether it's in a classroom or not.

DEMANDING IDENTITY

Tonight I was out in town with Ruth and Catherine who both have Tourettes. As soon as we got to the pub we were ID'd – not, sadly, to prove our ages, but to prove we had Tourettes.

The bar manager approached us while we were waiting to be served and stood in front of us for a long time, staring. Eventually he managed to say, 'I need to ask ...' but stumbled over his words, giggling nervously before finally getting it out, 'I have to ask, have you got a real condition or are you taking the piss?'

We explained we have Tourettes and he replied, 'I'm sorry, but I have to think of my other customers. Do you have proof?' Fortunately, we do all have ID cards that confirm we have Tourettes. He looked at Ruth's first, and then he studied mine for a long time. Finally, despite having seen both Ruth's and mine, he still insisted on seeing Catherine's.

He agreed to serve us but said, 'You need to keep it down.' We explained that it doesn't really work like that but he just repeated, 'You're going to offend my customers.'

We pointed out that we were his customers and that he was offending us.

MYSTERIOUS MARKS

As I was leaving work last night I noticed a horizontal scratch on my cheek that hadn't been there earlier. I've discovered several other mystery marks over the last few months in exactly the same place, but I have no idea how they're getting there.

I mentioned this to Fat Sister later. She looked at my face and said, 'You also have a black eye.' I didn't believe her and tried to wipe it away, thinking it was just some dirt. But after a careful scrub I conceded that it was indeed a black eye.

I hadn't got a clue how this happened. I bash my face a lot but I tend to know immediately if I've actually hurt myself. It's disconcerting not knowing how these injuries occur.

What was one black eye last night had turned into two by the time I woke up this morning. This means I'm faced with the re-emergence of an old dilemma: how and when do I explain my injuries to others? People don't always ask and I never know whether to say something or not. Now I have to go to work looking like a panda.

PHONE ON THE EDGE

Leftwing Idiot and I were hanging out at his flat this evening. The window next to us was open to let what little breeze there was into the room. I suddenly found myself trying to post my phone out of the window. Leftwing Idiot moved swiftly and took it out of my hand.

Once the immediate risk had been averted he very deliberately put the phone on the window ledge. It was very distracting for me because I kept thinking about throwing it out. He knew what I was thinking and it made us both laugh. After a few moments he put the phone safely out of reach in a drawer.

A number of friends have said they hate standing at the edge of high buildings or railway platforms because they start to obsess about jumping. This might make most people feel anxious, but doesn't mean they'll end up doing anything dangerous. I'm different only because I sometimes have a problem controlling this urge and end up doing the risky thing impulsively.

16 BPM

King Russell and I have just done a little experiment – the con-
clusion of which is that I'm currently running at 16 bpm (biscuits
per minute). If this is a consistent rate, it means I tic 'biscuit'
approximately 960 times an hour, or over 16,000 times a day
while I'm awake. This means that over the last year I've said biscuit nearly 6,000,000 times.

That's a lot of biscuits.

NOSI

NOSI stands for Non-Obscene Socially Inappropriate behaviour.
This might include, for example, making remarks about someone's height or weight. It can be a feature of Tourettes although
it's not something that's generally a problem for me.

This evening I encountered a shopkeeper whose comments
would definitely come into the NOSI category, although as far as
I'm aware there was no neurological explanation – he was just
being rude. On my way home I popped into a shop near the lair
with Leftwing Idiot. The shopkeeper asked him, 'What's wrong
with her body?' I assumed he meant my tics, but before I had a
chance to respond he said, 'Last year she was slimmer.'

I turned on him, snapping, 'Why would you ask him *that*?
Would you say that to any other woman who came into your
shop?' He apologised repeatedly and my anger faded slightly but
I left feeling upset and undermined.

Despite how unusually my body moves and the number of
people who comment on it, I don't feel particularly sensitive
most of the time. What really annoyed me about what he said
was that I'm sure he wouldn't have said it to a non-disabled
customer.

It wasn't just *my* body being judged today. Laura sent me a text later recounting a conversation she'd had with a colleague at work who'd told her being pregnant was no excuse for putting on weight!

STAYING STRONG, STAYING IN

PART ONE

It's a Saturday evening in the middle of summer. I haven't got any work commitments and I want to go and see what's happening in town.

Instead, I'm sitting in the lair on my own, half-watching Columbo.

I've wanted to go out and do something all afternoon, but except for a brief outing this morning to view a nearby flat, I haven't been out at all. My feeling of frustration is getting stronger as the evening slips by.

Previously I would've gone to an exhibition, for a look round the shops or for a walk on my own, but this is no longer possible because of my leg tics. I feel trapped and depressed.

Everything's made worse by the fact that my internet isn't working properly.

PART TWO

While I was writing I started to cry. I phoned Laura, we had a chat and I cried a bit more. But by the end of the call I felt more positive, and just then Poppy and Leftwing Idiot arrived at the lair. I was still feeling tearful but I went back with them to Leftwing Idiot's and we sat on his roof, ate banana ice cream and watched the sun set.

SPONTANEOUS SHAKESPEARE

It was just me at the lair this afternoon. I was doing some washing up and generally pottering about, when I suddenly and loudly ticced: 'It is the hippies of outrageous fortune that weigh heavy on the minds of dogs.'

Spontaneous Shakespeare on a Sunday afternoon is one of the joys of Tourettes.

AN EXPLOSION

It had started as a standout day. I'd been unusually still and my tics were much less intense than normal. But it didn't last. In the afternoon they suddenly and dramatically intensified, and once again I found myself stuck on the floor, unable to get up. I was at work and fortunately Leftwing Idiot was there to provide support. He made the area around me safe and held my head to stop it hitting the filing cabinets nearby. My body moved constantly for nearly an hour, contorting and jerking uncontrollably. The sensation was completely overpowering, like some sort of surging electric shock. Eventually, with the help of some diazepam, normal ticcing levels resumed.

Later, Leftwing Idiot asked me which I'd choose if I could: ticcing steadily all day, or having one concentrated burst and being calm for the rest of the time. I couldn't decide.

SOUNDS SENSITIVE

Leftwing Idiot and I dropped in on King Russell and Fat Sister in their new place earlier. We were sitting in the living room while King Russell constructed some new flat-pack furniture. I found the noise of the drill really difficult to tolerate. It made me squeal and I had to cover my ears. Not long after, it was King Russell who was squealing and covering his.

I started talking to Fat Sister about how I was going to have a long overdue smear test. King Russell can't cope with hearing any words associated with the vagina so this conversation was always going to be difficult for him.

Smear tests are unpleasant at the best of times, but my main worry's been about staying still long enough for it to be done and not over-reacting in the process. Discussing the practicalities of all this was more than King Russell could manage. He put down his drill and went to another room.

TIC SQUEAK

Although it's Sunday I was at work today because we had a big group of young volunteers who'd come to help out with some painting. At lunchtime I was sitting with a group of them whom I hadn't met before and they were very interested in the gloves I wear to protect my hands and chest from my banging tic.

This isn't unusual – I've had lots of curious and complimentary comments from kids about my gloves. But it turned out this group were intrigued because they thought the gloves had a squeaker inside them. I had to gently explain it was me squeaking, not the gloves!

WRIGGLY SPINE

I've talked a bit before about what my physical tics feel like, and while the sensation that comes with them is incredibly strong, I find it hard to describe. Tics often make my body contort dramatically. It feels a bit like suddenly being wrenched from the inside. Leftwing Idiot asked me the other day if the tics hurt. I wouldn't say they cause pain, but to describe it as discomfort doesn't convey their overwhelming strength.

At the moment I've got a particularly distressing tic in my back. It comes in sudden bursts with great force, making it impossible for me to keep still.

Sometimes this feeling overwhelms my whole body and it feels like someone's put itching powder in my blood. Other people can hold me to stop me hurting myself but they can't stop the sensation.

Even so, it's preferable to be held rather than end up with another black eye.

AUGUST

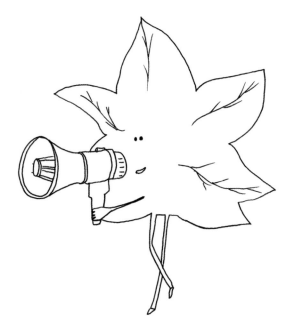

SOFTLY SPOKEN AUTUMN

RETURN OF THE GLOVE

August is one of the busiest months of the year where I work. All three of the children's projects I help run are in the middle of their summer holiday play schemes. Every day children are turning up to enjoy the sunshine and their freedom from school.

My leg tics are making it very difficult to get around at the moment, and seeing this, the children have been coming up with cunning solutions to help me out. One boy cycled me across the playground on a large two-seater tricycle and volunteered to be my taxi for the afternoon.

This wasn't the only helping hand I got at work. During the Easter holidays another younger boy nabbed one of my padded gloves and took it home. He'd been promising to return it ever since – and today he finally did, freshly laundered by his mum.

SUMMER STARE-OUT

I was lucky to be able to enjoy a funny conversation with a child at my work this afternoon.

We were sitting in the garden by the pond, shaded by a green canopy with patches of sun making their way through the leaves. The girl I was with is seven and together we were looking into the water and talking about what might live beneath the surface.

I said, 'We need to be quiet so we don't scare the fish,' but added, 'I'm not very good at being quiet.' She looked at me and said, 'I know why you can't be quiet. It's because you have to squeak.' I said, 'Yep, but I think the fish will get used to it.' She agreed and said, 'I have.'

I'd briefly explained Tourettes to her before, like I do with lots of children, but she went on to ask some thoughtful questions about what it felt like. I didn't mention my wriggly spine but instead I asked her what her body did all the time without her thinking about it.

She couldn't think of anything, so I pointed out how she blinked all the time. She laughed and said, 'If I don't blink it hurts, I have to blink.' I said, 'That's a bit like how it feels for me if I don't move or make a noise.'

She suggested we had a no blinking competition. 'Squeaking's OK, though,' she was careful to point out. We sat on the ground next to the pond in an amazing wild space and stared at each other. London's never felt so peaceful.

She won.

PASSING THE BISCUIT TEST

When I'm not very well my tics tend to reduce, both in frequency and intensity. It's as if my body recognises the need to conserve energy, so many of the tics become gentler and less complex as a result.

I've been under the weather for the last couple of days and, true to form, most of my verbal tics have calmed down a lot. They've also been harder to trigger.

Leftwing Idiot's been doing what he calls the 'Biscuit Test'. This involves him saying 'biscuit' to me in a way that would normally make me echo it back. While I've been ill this hasn't been happening, but that's not stopped him from trying.

He knew I was getting better today though when I passed the 'Biscuit Test' by energetically ticcing 'biscuit' back to him at top volume.

NEW LAIR

Today I bought a new lair. It's only a few minutes away from where I am now and even closer to Leftwing Idiot's. Crucially, it's on the ground floor, and has a garden. It was a daunting decision but one that will make a big difference to my independence, safety, and quality of life.

I've decided to rent out the old lair, so in just a few weeks time I'll move out and new tenants will move in. There's a lot to sort out before then, but I'm very excited and can't wait to live in a place where I can get to all the rooms safely and where I'm a lot less likely to get stranded inside on a sunny day.

It's a momentous occasion and as I sit and reflect on it I'm very aware of the mix of emotions I'm feeling. I'm:

    50% excited about having an amazing new place to live
    15% sad to leave the lair, a place where I've been very happy
        for a long time
    15% worried about the complicated and stressful process of
        moving
    20% relieved because soon I'll be in a place where getting to
        my clothes doesn't involve dicing with death on the stairs

This move is only happening because of the support and assistance of my friends and family. I'm aiming for 100% good times with them all in the new lair.

'WHO WANTS A WHISKEY?'

I went for a long-awaited trip to the dentist this afternoon. It was with the special care team at my local hospital. I'd been referred to them because my tics have become too difficult for my existing dentist to manage.

Leftwing Idiot came with me, and while we were sitting in the waiting room an older woman walked in and started talking to the receptionist. We both noticed she was wearing a Blue Peter badge. I fought to control my tics but didn't manage it for long:

'I've got a Blue Peter badge in Pig Porn.'
'Hands up if you've got a ship on you.'

The woman didn't seem to notice and luckily my name was soon called out to go through. The dentist, his assistant and two dental nurses were lovely, welcoming and reassuring. My old dentist had said he felt I needed to be sedated, but the specialist wanted to see if laughing gas would be sufficient to subdue my tics, because if it did it would make future treatment much easier.

I breathed the gas in through a mask with the dentist gradually increasing the amount of nitrous oxide, but I carried on moving and making noises with the same force. He kept asking how I felt and my answer didn't change: 'Relaxed, but I don't think I'm any stiller.' After several increases, my tics became less complex and I started making the loud squawk I often make when I'm going to sleep. But I was still moving about a lot.

In spite of this, they decided to have a go at examining and cleaning my teeth. The dental nurse held my forehead and Leftwing Idiot held my hands and legs.

During the course of cleaning one of my fillings came out, which was an extra problem they had to fix.

I continued to tic throughout the treatment:

'Who likes Dizzy Rascal?'
'Who wants a whiskey?'

They all laughed and the dentist said, 'I'll definitely need a glass of wine this evening.'

At one point I started to feel horrible, like I was going to pass out. I managed to indicate that I wasn't OK and that I felt very heavy. They stopped the gas and gave me pure oxygen instead.

We did the rest of the treatment the old fashioned way, without gas, and with Leftwing Idiot and the dental team holding me down. The dentist fixed my broken filling, which looks a lot better than it did before.

The whole process lasted about an hour and I was very relieved when it was over. When it was all done the dentist said, 'We won't do it that way again.'

I'm guessing he's well into his second glass of wine by now.

♥ # %

My tics appear to be experimenting with symbols. Hearts, hashtags and percentages have all recently featured. Here are a handful of symbolic examples:

'I ♥ cum.'
'#pickledonioncumbottle.'
'I'm 40% more biscuity than sheep.'
'I ♥ robot legs.'
'#teacuptits.'
'95% of biscuits are birds.'

SWIMMING NOT DROWNING

This afternoon Poppy and I went swimming at the local pool. I haven't been for ages and it was a bit of an experiment, inspired by my brief swim in Cornwall.

The lifeguard was amazingly helpful. Poppy asked her for a hand while I got ready and both of them helped me get safely to the edge of the pool. I'd been worrying about this for a while before we got there.

Getting in was easy and I managed to swim much better than I'd expected. The great thing about swimming is the support the water gives my body. When I tic it slows my movements right down and it doesn't take long for me to sort myself out. It did involve swallowing half the pool though, because my vocal tics didn't stop when I was underwater.

I swam close to the edge with Poppy alongside me. She said, 'The only bit that makes me nervous is when your head goes under.' And she was quick to provide help when it did.

Keeping moving took a lot of concentration and I got tired quickly, but it was very invigorating. Nobody seemed at all bothered by my noisy swimming style, even when every so often I helpfully shouted, 'I'm drowning!'

WHEELS?

Leftwing Idiot and I were talking about my walking today. It's been getting steadily worse over the last few months so we discussed whether using a wheelchair might be a good idea. Neither of us could decide one way or another, so I've made a list of pros and cons to see if it makes things clearer:

Pros
Less risk of causing injury or strain to the person helping me
Less risk of injuring my knees, ankles, or head, or falling down, especially in the road
Not so tiring for me and the person helping me
Greater freedom in getting around

Cons
Less exercise for me, which is already limited by my tics
I'd need strapping in thoroughly to make sure I didn't jump out

Some people would see it as a step backwards – less
   independence not more

It would take up extra space

That hasn't made it any clearer. The more I think about it the more complicated it becomes. I don't think using a wheelchair would make me any more or any less independent because I already need help to move around safely. It might make longer journeys much easier, and the idea of using a chair in certain situations is very appealing. But I don't want to give in to the tics or become less active.

My thoughts are muddled and I'm finding it hard to pick apart what I think is best for me, my concerns for those who support me, and my worry about what other people might think.

DIDN'T SHE DO WELL?

The radio was on in the cab on the way to work this morning. It's GCSE results day and young people were being interviewed about how well they'd done. As usual the presenter was going on about how much easier the exams are these days and how illiterate young people have become. People were phoning in and offering much the same opinions. It's the same thing every year.

Several hours later I ticced my own results:

'I have a GCSE in lungs.'
'I have fourteen GCSEs in crime.'
'I have a GCSE in addiction to crisps.'
'I have an A* in botulism.'
'I have a GCSE in mums.'
'I don't have a GCSE in Christmas.'

We'll just have to see how far I get with these credentials.

IN THE WORDS OF MY TEACHERS

The other day Leftwing Idiot said, 'I'd love to have met you as a kid – what were you like?' Today, while we were sorting out mountains of paperwork at the old lair, I was able to tell him, in the words of my primary school teachers. Here's what they wrote in my reports:

'A bundle of bouncy energy. She does not seem to mind making an exhibition of herself.'

'There are signs that she is becoming more calm. However her rather scatty personality, however endearing, has restricted her progress.'

'Generally speaking a well-behaved child yet she can become quite aggressive e.g. pinching, pushing.'

'She is unable to sit still for very long and is constantly on the move, with, at times, unfortunate results: Falling off chairs, tripping over.'

'A naturally creative child. Her paintings and drawings are lively and colourful and have a certain style to them, even though they appear a little messy. Her work is quite individualistic.'

'She is an intelligent, articulate and active child but can be uncoordinated and has difficulty with manipulating cutlery.'

'A great sense of humour, common sense and enthusiasm.'

'We continue to work on her motor control and body awareness.'

'She has been arriving at school with a little more composure recently which is a good sign.'

'Specific speech therapy has been aimed at stopping the dribbling she finds a problem. She should be proud of her achievement in learning to eat and drink in a way that looks normal.'

So now he knows.

RAPID RESPONSE

This morning I had my needs assessed by a social worker from the Physical Disabilities Team. She was friendly, listened carefully and took time to understand my situation. It was a relief to talk about the impact my tics have on my life with someone who can provide some actual resources to help.

To my amazement, she got in touch a few hours later to tell me a temporary package of support had already been approved. To start with this will be provided by a care agency, but longer term I'll get a personal budget and I'll be able to employ a support worker to help me at home.

This evening I've been thinking about what to include in my support plan. I hope the additional help will take a little bit of the pressure off my friends and family and give me the freedom to plan and make decisions independently.

I feel hopeful.

SEPTEMBER

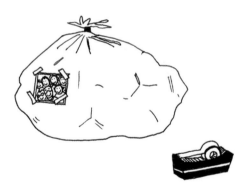

I   SELLOTAPED MY LIFE TO A BIN BAG.

THE DYING FISH

While I was having a shower this morning, I started ticcing inten-
sively. For safety I always shower sitting down but the tics meant
I'd slipped right down and I started what Leftwing Idiot refers to
as my dying fish move. This is a fairly accurate description for the
abrupt backwards and forwards movement of my body when I'm
horizontal and ticcing.

The complication of doing the dying fish in the bath is that
there's not much room, so I kept banging my head, arms and legs
on the side. The shower hurtling water straight into one ear
didn't help much, and as the water pooled around my face I
thought, 'Uh oh!'

The whole thing was distressing and frightening, but eventually I managed to roll onto my back, pull myself up and get out.

If I'm going to stop myself dying in the bath I need to find a
better solution for when this fishy little move happens.

SAFE START

Leftwing Idiot and Poppy headed off for a long-awaited holiday
first thing this morning. I've just had a text to say they've had a
smooth journey and have arrived safely.

I had a smooth start to my day too, and arrived at work feeling unusually serene. This is because the carer my social worker
has organised for me started today.

The carer's lovely. I'd been worried it would be a different
person every day, but she assured me she'll be my regular carer.

Having her help made getting ready for work much easier, and
things which had begun to feel like an extreme sport are now a
little bit safer.

SO LONG, STAIRS

This will be my last night at the old lair. It's been my home for four years and I've always enjoyed living here, but in the last six months it's become increasingly difficult to manage the six flights of stairs because of my leg tics.

A year ago I wouldn't have predicted I'd have to move out because of my tics, and it's strange to think my body's made that decision for me against my will.

Although I feel a tinge of sadness, I'm relieved that tonight's climb up to my front door will be the last in a long while. All I have to do now is get safely down again tomorrow, and then it's 'So long, stairs.'

GERANIUM EVACUATION

I moved out of the lair today and into Leftwing Idiot's flat, where I'll be staying for a few weeks before moving into my new super-hero home. Leftwing Idiot isn't here – he's on holiday with Poppy. Something else very familiar has also gone – the geranium. I've got a strange obsession with this plant and since its arrival in Leftwing Idiot's kitchen a few months ago I've kept making rude comments about it and swearing at it.

Before he went away Leftwing Idiot took the geranium all the way across town to his parents because he didn't trust me with it. Personally I don't think this was necessary, although this evening I did tic, 'I've got the kill-a-geranium virus.'

MY HEAD'S SPINNING

My cab driver told me this morning that I was 'possessed'. He said I should ask a priest for help. I told him that I didn't feel very possessed and that I'm generally quite nice to people. I asked him why, if an evil spirit had taken my soul, it would make me shout about biscuits. He couldn't give me an answer.

It might be hard to believe but this isn't the first time a cab driver's suggested I might have fallen victim to demonic possession. A while ago I went to a party in Clapham for Laura's birthday and travelled home with my friend Emma in a black cab. We dropped her off first then headed for the lair. As we pulled up, the driver said, 'Exorcism would cure you,' and we talked for a while about his belief that I was possessed.

I tried pointing out some of the problems with his arguments but gave up after he said that if I didn't have an exorcism the evil spirit would get worse and I'd end up with cerebral palsy.

DISTURBING HAIR DAY

Shopkeeper: 'Are you disturbed?'
   TH: 'No, I have Tourettes Syndrome. I'm not disturbed.'
   Shopkeeper: 'What about your hair?'

WHAT GOES BUMP IN THE NIGHT?

Me. In the early hours this morning I got stuck doing the dying fish in Leftwing Idiot's hallway. I was worrying about two main things as I struggled to regain control and get up:

1) The noise of my head banging on the floor disturbing his neighbours
2) Getting blood on his carpet

Fortunately I was able to get up reasonably quickly, and the tiny spot of blood wiped off easily too, so I needn't have worried. When I looked in the mirror I saw an imprint of the carpet on my forehead, so it was the carpet that'd left its mark on me. This made me laugh, but not loud enough to disturb the neighbours.

ROBOT, DRUM OR DOG?

I'm always interested in how children react to and understand my tics. I'm very aware when explaining Tourettes that I need to be clear and accurate without worrying or confusing them.

This afternoon at work I spent a lot of time playing with a boy of about three who was visiting the playground with his mum and siblings. He was a bit young for a verbal explanation but nevertheless seemed unfazed by my tics. To start with, every time I banged my chest he would tap his own or reach out and tap mine. But he soon forgot about this and became more absorbed by the games we were playing. Another child said that I was 'a bit like a robot because you don't control your body'.

I enjoy hearing children put Tourettes into new contexts because it makes me think about it in different ways. I've also been compared to an animated dog in a recent children's film.

TICCING BOMB

While I was waiting for a train today with my friend Bunny I found myself shouting 'Bomb!' (among other things). Rather inevitably, a policeman who'd been standing nearby marched over to us.

Policeman: Do you think that's a sensible word to be shouting?
TH: No, obviously not, but I can't stop it.
Policeman: Of course you can.
TH: I have Tourettes Syndrome so I really can't.
Policeman: Well I'm just telling you that if you say that word and a member of the public tells us, certain things will happen.

TH: I understand that and wouldn't choose to say it. But I have to trust that most people will see it's just one of the many words I can't stop myself saying.

He looked at Bunny and said, 'I've seen a bit of Tourettes but never as much as *this*.'

'KEITH DUFFY'S ALLERGIC TO PEANUTS'

Out of the blue today I ticced 'Keith Duffy's allergic to peanuts'.

Keith was a member of '90s pop sensations Boyzone. To be clear, I've got no particular interest in Boyzone, or in celebrity gossip, or allergies, so I assumed this was just a typical tic, splicing together different ideas with no basis in reality.

On a whim this evening I went online to check if he *was* allergic to peanuts. To my surprise there were a number of articles confirming that he was. This isn't recent news, and I don't remember ever having seen or heard anything about it.

This leads me to conclude there are three possible explanations:

1) It's a complete coincidence
2) I'm magic
3) I'd seen a reference to his allergy in passing at some point and Tourettes decided today was the day to share this fragment of information from deep inside my mind.

I hope this information proves useful should you find yourself planning snack options for a Boyzone reunion concert.

A HELPING HAND WHEN I NEED IT

When I got up to get some water in the early hours this morning I was ticcing a lot and I dropped down in Leftwing Idiot's kitchen.

My body was moving and twisting all over the place and I couldn't get back up. This has happened before, and when I'm on my own it often takes a long time before I regain control. But now Poppy and Leftwing Idiot are back from their holiday I'm no longer alone. Leftwing Idiot heard the sound of the chairs banging against the table and came to help me get back to bed.

Ticcing in the middle of the night has often left me feeling trapped and frightened. It's been amazing since I came to stay at Leftwing Idiot's, knowing that someone's always around and listening out for me. But I'm only staying here for a few weeks, and when I'm in my new place I won't have this sort of help. It's another thing to worry about, but for the moment I'm just appreciating the help and the peace of mind it brings me.

'HELLO BASIL, YOU LOOK FRESH'

Poppy brought a new plant home this evening. Unlike the geranium (which for its own safety is still at Leftwing Idiot's parents' house), my tics seem to have taken an instant shine to the basil plant.

After a careful inspection of the newly arrived herb I announced, 'I tenderly fucked a basil plant.'

I'm not sure what Mr Otter will make of this new love interest but we'll cross that bridge when we come to it.

TOURETTES AND LOVING IT

Online I often come across comments about Tourettes such as: 'Why do people with Tourettes Syndrome say only bad things?' or, 'Why don't you get any cases of nice Tourettes?'

My newest tic clearly shows Tourettes can be very nice indeed: I've started ticcing 'I love you.'

It's friendly but a bit confusing. If I were saying 'I hate you', I'd expect my family and friends to recognise it was a tic, and that

I didn't mean it. But with this new one, sometimes I *do* love the people I'm saying it to, and while I haven't *chosen* to say it, I don't want them to hear it as just a tic.

That said, I'm randomly declaring my love to strangers, colleagues and a variety of inanimate objects as well.

STAND AND DELIVER

I went into the post office this morning and as I approached the counter I shouted, 'Hands up!'

Fortunately I'm a regular customer so this didn't result in any panic buttons being pressed.

Getting to know people in shops and cafes I visit regularly is very important to me. It makes me feel safe in the knowledge that they know who I am, and why I'm talking and moving in the way I do.

I reckon, for a lot of people with Tourettes, how happy and secure they feel where they live extends beyond their immediate friends and family into the wider local community.

So this morning I was able to post my letter without fear of arrest, and that feels very good indeed.

HEARING BISCUITS

Fat Sister told me that yesterday, during the night shift at the hospital where she works, one of the nurses was offering people biscuits. She kept saying, 'Biscuit?' 'Biscuit?' 'Biscuit?' Fat Sister started laughing because she found it so odd to hear this incredibly familiar word without me being around.

The nurse asked why she was laughing and she explained. Apparently this made all the nurses laugh, but then they looked a bit guilty and said they were sorry. 'You don't need to apologise,' she said, 'it can be very funny.'

Fat Sister's not the only person hearing biscuits. My friend Hannah, who's a fashion designer in charge of colour samples, says she thinks of me every time anyone asks for the 'biscuit-coloured' sample. Leftwing Idiot did a double take when a decorator started talking about 'biscuit tiles'. When Poppy was working late into the night recently her colleague shouted out for a biscuit, which she found very amusing for the same reason.

I'm glad to know my biscuits are rubbing off on the people around me.

FIGHTING THE FIREPLACE

It's Leftwing Idiot's birthday and he's already had three special birthday meals – breakfast and tea, then dinner this evening with Poppy. While they were out I was in his flat on my own, working on the computer and enjoying a relaxing evening. I got up to get something from the other room and after a few faltering steps I dropped to the floor in the kitchen.

Leftwing Idiot has beautiful old fireplaces and it was one of these – and his tiled floor – that my hands hit repeatedly at full force. I was on the floor for about ten minutes before I managed to push myself into a safe sitting position. By then my wrists were bruised and swollen.

When I'd first got up from the computer I hadn't put my gloves on. I'd taken them off to type and didn't bother to put them back on because I'd thought I'd only be standing for a minute. If I had been wearing gloves, my hands wouldn't have got damaged.

Once I'd managed to sit up, it felt safest to stay where I was rather than risk trying to go anywhere and getting into trouble again. So I sat on the floor and waited for Leftwing Idiot and Poppy to get back.

They came home about half an hour later and quickly helped me clean and ice my hands. As soon as they got in I started to shake with shock – I felt embarrassed and annoyed with myself that they'd come home to find me trembling and crying on the kitchen floor.

The fact is, I could've taken some simple precautions to prevent these injuries. I've decided that when I'm on my own I'll make sure I'm properly kitted out when I'm moving about. I'm going to put a sign up to remind myself.

Alone? Getting Up? Walking?
1) Put padded gloves on
2) Put on or pull up knee pads
3) Put your phone in your pocket

After the ice my wrists felt better, and after a cup of tea and some time spent sitting round the kitchen table chatting *I* felt better too.

OCTOBER

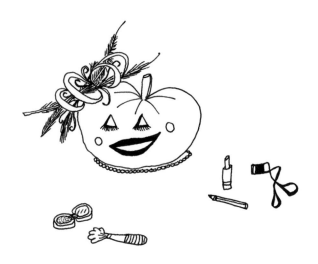

HELLO OCTOBER YOU'RE LOOKING SEXY.

'HELLO OCTOBER, YOU'RE LOOKING SEXY'

Poppy and I went out for dinner together tonight. On our walk back we had a seasonally appropriate discussion.

TH: I'm not a big fan of autumn.
Poppy: I am. I love autumn, me.
TH: Well you don't have such an intimate relationship with it as I do.
Poppy: I suppose between your hair, your gloves and your kneepads you do get quite leafy.

At which point she reached forward and pulled a twig out of my hair.

MY NEW LAIR

The new lair officially became mine today. I picked up the keys this afternoon and along with Bunny and Poppy headed off to let myself in for the first time. We bought smoothies from a nearby café and sat on the living room floor to enjoy them. The room was glowing with autumn sunlight as we chatted about what furniture we needed and how it could all be arranged. I felt instantly happy and at home there.

The building's an old pub which, as I know from having lived in the area for a long time, has had a colourful past. After years of dereliction following two rather suspicious fires it's been turned into flats, and I've got one on the ground floor.

All the rooms have lovely high ceilings and big windows, making it feel spacious and light throughout. If I sound like an estate agent it's because I'm very excited about the prospect of living here.

The living room's double doors open onto a huge private courtyard that's almost as big as the flat itself. I'll be able to sit out there whenever I want, which will make getting stuck inside on hot days a thing of the past.

There are two bedrooms. The bigger one will be mine and the other will be Poppy's. We're not moving in straightaway, though – we're going to stay at Leftwing Idiot's until we've bought everything we need for living in this amazing place.

Although I've looked round it several times before, being here today felt different. I've spent the last few months imagining life in my new home, so knowing it's actually mine now is brilliant. I've been noticing small details which I know will become important to me, like the row of majestic trees I can see from my bedroom or the windowsill in the kitchen that makes a perfect place to sit.

Besides the obvious advantages of not having stairs to worry about, there are lots of other things about my new home that'll make life much easier. I heard Poppy describing it as 'Tourettes-friendly' to King Russell. He said, 'So it's got squashy carpets and soft-close drawers, then?'

He was right, it has.

SWEARING AT MYSELF

I have copropraxia, which means I tic rude gestures. More specifically, I have a habit of sticking my finger up at anything. I've done it to Leftwing Idiot's geranium, the TV, light fittings, random passers-by and my friend Hannah's fourteen-month-old son. Recently I've taken to swearing at the whole room by sticking my finger up and panning through 180 degrees.

Tonight, having sworn at everything else, I started sticking my fingers up at each other!

COVENTRY -- CITY OF SILENCE

Coventry, a city usually associated with silence, got a taste of the noisy treatment today as it hosted a conference on Tourettes.

Leftwing Idiot, Ruth and I travelled there by train. The air conditioning was on full blast in our carriage and Ruth kept ticcing 'HELP! I'm cold.' We reached Coventry unusually chilly, but in good time and made our way to the massive Methodist church where the conference was being held. We joined many other people with Tourettes, and their families, who'd come from all over the UK to hear about the latest research and to socialise and share experiences.

A conference full of lots of people with Tourettes is a strange affair and there were plenty of funny moments. One person's tics would start someone else's off, forming chains of tics around the room. At my table we had an outbreak of counting out loud, and at one point at least five of us were meowing like cats.

A mother whose son has Tourettes said, 'You have to get a sense of humour when you get a diagnosis of Tourettes.'

The event was attended by people of all ages and this gave it a really warm atmosphere. I liked the mixture of adults, parents, children, teenagers, partners and friends. I felt relaxed being somewhere my behaviour was understood and didn't stand out.

On the train home I was pulled back to reality when the ticket inspector, pointing at me, said to Leftwing Idiot, 'Does the woman have a problem?' He said, 'You should ask her.' Ruth was impressed by how Leftwing Idiot handled the situation. When she'd had a similar experience, the friend she'd been with had been embarrassed and hadn't known how to react.

RAGE

At the conference last weekend one of the speakers discussed rage attacks, which is the term for sudden, out-of-control, explosive outbursts that happen without warning. Rage attacks are associated with Tourettes in some people. I've seen them described as the release of tension that's been building up, and they're usually followed by feelings of intense remorse.

When I was a child my behaviour could be wildly unpredictable. I would enter what my dad described as a 'black hole' and I'd become angry and distressed. This sometimes included lashing out at other people or breaking things. My parents' house still bears some of the scars of these episodes. I didn't feel in control when they happened and I can remember knowing what was happening, but not being able to find a way to calm down. I'd feel horrible and very guilty afterwards.

I grew out of this and I'm generally much calmer these days. Even so, I sometimes find it difficult to manage extremes of emotion because my tics, and my frustration with them, intensify at these times. It's a feeling reminiscent of how I felt as a child.

Leftwing Idiot hadn't heard about rage attacks until the other weekend. But since then he's been enjoying asking me if I'm about to have a rage attack whenever I show the slightest hint of frustration about anything.

FUCKING GOATS, CHUCKING BALLS

Today, Leftwing Idiot pointed out how handy it is he's got a good sense of humour. He's quite right – some people might find a conversation like the one we just had insulting and certainly not, as he found it, hilarious.

LI: I've got to …
TH: Fuck a goat.
LI: OK, not that. I've got to …
TH: Fuck a goat.
Poppy: What have you got to do?
TH: Fuck a goat.

This went on without stopping for quite a while until eventually we found out what Leftwing Idiot had to do.

My interruptions and impulsive behaviour have sometimes got me into trouble. I suddenly remembered an occasion at school during a joint PE lesson with another class. We were sitting in lines with our teacher in front of us. He told everyone to put their basketball down on the floor. And that's what everyone else did. I, however, picked mine up and threw it with full force straight at him.

There was a big gasp and a ripple of nervous laughter when it hit him square in the face. He immediately ordered me out of the gym.

I was terrified and very shocked by what I'd done. He came out and told me off, but I remember being surprised at how lenient and understanding he was and how he accepted my explanation that it had 'just happened'.

WHO'S WORRIED?

When I phoned the bank this afternoon I explained to the person who answered that I had Tourettes. And she said, 'That's OK I don't mind, don't worry about it.'

Although she meant this to sound positive, whenever anyone says something like that it gives me a jolt. It happens quite a lot and feels like my explanation has been understood as an apology. I'd prefer people to say something like, 'Thanks for telling me.'

I don't tell people I've got Tourettes because I think they'll mind, and I wouldn't expect them to be worried by it either. The reason I tell them is so they understand and don't get confused by all the 'biscuits'.

I HAVEN'T SPOKEN ABOUT SPEAKING

I've had a difficult time today. I've had a series of extreme, explosive ticcing episodes which have meant that my body has been completely taken over by continuous motor tics. Typically these episodes have lasted about half an hour and they've left me feeling totally exhausted.

I've had episodes like this before every now and again (I'd refer to it as doing the dying fish), but never as many times in one day. They started out of the blue this morning, with no obvious triggers. I'm very lucky that Leftwing Idiot's been with me all day and has kept me safe.

A new development is that I'm also finding it hard to speak. This has happened on other occasions recently, and not just during these very extreme ticcing periods. I know exactly what I want to say but it feels like my tics block the words from forming and all that comes out is a strange dinosaur-like screech or a jumble of noises.

Naturally I'm finding all this quite alarming, but I also know I'm being well supported and I've coped with frightening shifts in my tics like this before. I'm hoping today was a one-off or at least very unusual, but if it's not I know that with help I'll find a way of managing.

SLEEPING IT OFF

I've spent much more time asleep than awake today because of some drugs I was given last night to stop me ticcing.

The explosive ticcing episodes I described a couple of days ago carried on yesterday. Leftwing Idiot and I agreed that if my tics went on unbroken for more than 30 minutes, and if the emergency medication I have at home failed to work, he'd call an ambulance. They did go on for longer than that and the medication didn't work, so late in the evening he called for help.

We'd agreed all this in advance, but I'd warned him I might disagree when it came to it and that I might ask him not to call an ambulance. In the event I knew I needed help and agreed instantly with his decision.

The team at the hospital were amazing, and they were eventually able to calm my tics down to normal levels using a combination of drugs. While we were waiting for these to take effect a nurse and medical student helped Leftwing Idiot keep me safe by holding me on the thin hospital bed. After about an hour of this, Leftwing Idiot noticed the medical student looked uncomfortable and it turned out he'd been on his way to the toilet when I came in and he'd wanted to go ever since. But like a true professional he'd diligently stayed and held onto my wriggling body until we told him it was all right to go. At least there was one less person wriggling.

At one stage I remember shouting, 'Help! I'm stuck down a well!' and hearing Leftwing Idiot explain to the nurse that I wasn't panicking and knew exactly where I was.

I wasn't the only one shouting in the ward last night. An elderly Irish man in the next bay was busy swearing angrily at the medical staff. Each time he swore my tics echoed back. The nurse holding my arms said he was quieter than he'd been all evening after I arrived.

Once the drugs had taken effect we came back home. The combination of the medication and the exertion of sustained ticcing meant that I haven't been able to do very much today other than sleep.

WHEN 'THANK-YOU'S' GO BAD

Of all my vocal tics, if I could lose just two I'd choose 'Thank you' and 'Sorry'. This might sound strange, but 'Thank you' and 'Sorry' only come up as tics when I'm feeling insecure. They've become an automatic reaction to feeling worried or guilty about the help I'm being given or the distress or bother other tics have caused.

These words are important to me and I want to be in control of when I use them, but ticcing them repeatedly devalues not only the words themselves but also the generosity of the help or support I'm being given. It's also very annoying. Sorry.

FIGHTING MUM

My mum and I generally have a peaceful relationship, but out of nowhere this evening I started ticcing a long and complex poem about fighting her. It was spilling out of my mouth much faster than Leftwing Idiot could write, so most of it got lost. But he did manage to capture this stanza:

'I'll fight my mum in Spandex,
I'll fight my mum in Rome,
I'll fight my mum in Hampstead Heath,
And in Kwik Fit on Roman Road.'

I'm a long way off poet laureate standard, but it's a start.

WHO'S 'IT'?

I went for an appointment at the National Hospital for Neurology and Neurosurgery today, with Leftwing Idiot. When we arrived we sat in the main waiting area and after a few minutes a member of staff came and said to him, 'Shall we put it in the corridor, so she's nearer her doctor?'

Leftwing Idiot didn't answer and indicated she should speak directly to me. This isn't the first time I've been encouraged to wait somewhere out of the way, but I've never been called 'it' before.

As we got out of the cab home tonight the driver leant over and said, 'The people who appear mad are often the most sane – it's the people trying to be normal who are crazy.'

I can try and take some encouragement from that at least.

BREAKING THE CODE

I've mentioned the difficulty I've been having speaking recently during these intense ticcing fits. It happened again today when I was with Fat Sister and King Russell. Fat Sister looked at me blankly each time I couldn't get the right words out – she had no idea what I was trying to say.

King Russell on the other hand managed to sort out whatever was on my mind and translate it perfectly. He's the only person I know who can make sense of the jumble of noises and words that come out of my mouth when I can't say what I'm trying to. He seems able to recognise something in their structure or content, link it all to what's going on around us, and then decode it.

It's an uncanny, baffling skill. Leftwing Idiot's explanation: 'He's a computer.'

SO MANY LAYERS OF SHIT

Last night I cried – I properly sobbed. It happened while I was talking to Leftwing Idiot about the acute ticcing fits I've been having over the past week. He said, 'You can't go into another week pretending everything's OK, because it's not.' I started to realise I have to face up to the knock-on implications of what's been happening. These fits affect:

My job
Leftwing Idiot's job
Moving into the new lair
My independence
and
My friends and family

I'm in a shit situation and feel overwhelmed by the many layers of interconnected shittiness. I'd been desperately hoping this would all stop, and while it still may, I now recognise I've got to start working on a plan for if it doesn't.

The first stage of this is to have some honest conversations with my boss, my social worker and my consultant.

I took the first step this morning when my boss came round to Leftwing Idiot's and we discussed the situation and made a plan for the week. I'm taking a couple of days off to recover some energy and to give me enough time to get in touch with all the other people and agencies involved in my care.

I know I can't put off getting in touch with Access to Work any longer. At the moment they fund a support worker for just two days a week, but if I'm to be able to keep working safely this will have to increase. Up to now I've been reluctant to ask for more help because I've been afraid that in the current climate they might cut what I get at the moment, and that would make work-ing impossible.

I feel much better now I've talked things through with my boss. She and all my colleagues are amazingly supportive and that's made me feel more optimistic than I was last night. I'm waiting to talk to my social worker next week, when she returns from holiday.

I'm beginning to sort out all the layers of this complicated situation, and I'm recognising the need to set up a comprehensive and holistic support system.

I've just got to work hard to make sure it all happens.

NOVEMBER

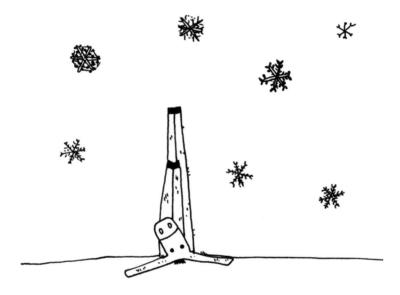

THIS IS THE WINTER OF YOUR DONKEY DOING HEADSTANDS.

A SUPPORTED START

Today my social worker presented my proposed individual budget and support plan to the panel that decides whether or not they will fund it. She also explained the impact the new ticcing fits are having on my life.

I'm relieved to say the panel agreed the plan. They also agreed some additional support overnight and at weekends, which will be reviewed next month.

I haven't been left alone since the ticcing fits intensified almost three weeks ago. Looking back, it's clear they began in July when I started getting stuck on the floor. Since they started happening several times a day, Leftwing Idiot's been providing most of the support and care I need. The new plan will mean I can employ personal assistants and carers so Leftwing Idiot and I can both regain some independence.

The support plan isn't the only line of attack on the ticcing fits – I'm also trying a medical intervention. In addition to the current medication, I'm going to try a drug I've not used before aimed at reducing the frequency of the attacks in the first place. I should know within a week or two if this is having a positive effect.

Previously, regular medication has either stopped working over time or the side effects have been more debilitating than the tics themselves. But I recognise that I'm now in an extreme situation and need to give new options try.

Over the last week the incredible responsiveness of the agencies supporting me has made me feel much more positive about the future. I've started to think about moving into my new lair again.

I'D DO ANYTHING

Here's my version of 'I'd do Anything' from the musical *Oliver!*. It came from nowhere this evening and is presented here verbatim (almost):

'I'd do anything for fucking mums, bitches and dog poo tits.
I'd do anything for a caged monkey in Peru.
I'd do anything for one last chance at Scrabble.
I'd do anything for Michael Jackson's mum to raise me up.
I'd do anything for Daz to really work.
I'd do anything for one basic human right to be over.
I'd do anything for toes made of butter.
I'd do anything for you Christmas pie.
I'd do anything for you Barbara Windsor.
I'd do anything for one night with David Dimbleby.
Yes, I'd do anything for you pisshead. Fuck off.
I'd climb a tree,
Paint your bumblebee (with ink made of tortoise spit).
Would you climb a tree?
No.
Paint your face bright blue?
Maybe, maybe not.
Visit China?
Maybe.
Visit Dagenham?
No.
I'd do anything for you, pisshead, pisshead, pisshead.
I'd climb a tree with my legs tied together, but not marry David
    Blunkett.
I'd do one thing now, and one thing later.
I'd do anything for larger breasts made of syrup.
Don't talk about syrup tits.
I'd do anything.

Anything?
Anything.
For one night of satisfaction with a revolver.
Put it on my tab.
I'd do anything except elongate my body.
I'd do anything for an imagination.
Would you climb Taylor Swift's underwear?
Talk to a Brazilian in Chinese?
I'd do anything for you to talk about fish.
I'd do a little bit for you dear, a little bit.
Anything for you!'

LIT UP BY LONDONERS

Tonight the sky's been lit up with fireworks. Like millions of other people across the city, we went off to a big organised display to celebrate Guy Fawkes Night. Naturally, my tics had organised a seasonal celebration of their own:

'Guy Fawkes is in my pants. Bang!'
'Roman Catholic Catherine wheels.'
'Guy Fawkes died. Bang!'

The council-funded display was amazing. It must've cost a bomb, and at a time when local authorities are under pressure to cut costs some people might argue against spending money on events like this. But there were thousands of people out to enjoy themselves and it was great to share something exciting and magical with so many other people.

The ticcing fits I've been having for the last few weeks have been dominating my life and restricting what I've been able to do, so it was with some trepidation that Leftwing Idiot, Poppy, and I set out this evening.

When we got to the park we made our way towards the

barriers. The crowd was already at least five people deep, but when Leftwing Idiot explained that I couldn't stand very well, we were let through to the front so I could hold the rail. To my left were a little girl and her mum whom I knew from work and to our right was a woman Leftwing Idiot and I had met on a course a few years ago. Even in a big crowd we were surrounded by friendly faces.

When the spectacular display had finished, there was the logistical nightmare of getting all 50,000 people through one set of tiny gates. Though we waited for some time, it still looked as if getting out safely would be impossible because I find it hard to stand still and move erratically at best.

Leftwing Idiot went and spoke to a steward who understood the problem very quickly. When he saw how tricky it was for me to walk, he let us through the barriers to use the crowd-free side. We still had to go through the same gates to get out, but he helped us by asking people to move out the way. Without his assistance we might have ended up in a dangerous situation.

As we approached the bus stop I began to have a ticcing fit. This wasn't ideal because we were on a crowded pavement by a busy road. But Leftwing Idiot and Poppy followed the plan I have for when this happens and they kept me safe. Poppy kept an eye out for any passing cabs, and it wasn't long before she spotted one and flagged it down. Many drivers, seeing a young woman writhing around on the pavement on a Saturday night, would've assumed I was drunk and refused to take me, but this driver didn't hesitate or even ask any questions. And by the time we got home I'd fully recovered. When Leftwing Idiot went to pay he refused to accept any money even though we tried to insist.

I've heard people say 'Community is dead' and that London is an unfriendly city. But tonight I felt very much part of my community and I was moved by the kindness and generosity of many people, both friends and strangers.

A MOMENT OF STILLNESS

One small good thing about ticcing fits is when they stop they leave me absolutely still for a few moments. This is the only time when I ever feel fully motionless. Then normal ticcing levels resume.

The fits are horrible, but the tiny moments of stillness are very precious and I find myself looking forward to them while I'm mid-writhe.

If I'm having a particularly bad time, Leftwing Idiot often tells me, 'This will pass.' He's right of course and I remind myself I've got some stillness to look forward to when it does.

STOP SNAPPING

My biting tics come and go, but even when they're not happening often, they're lurking in the background. They tend to flare up when I'm particularly upset, excited, angry or even happy, and although they can be triggered by strong emotions, they're still just tics over which I have little or no control.

What I do have is some control over the feelings that set the tics going. But, just like with anyone else, it's not always that easy to exert that control.

When Leftwing Idiot and I were arguing about something today I bit myself, so raising his voice in response he snapped, 'Stop it.' I understood completely why he did this (it must be very difficult to see me hurt myself like that), but my initial reaction was one of annoyance – if I could stop it, I would!

His reaction made me feel even more frustrated, but it's also made me make more of an effort to manage my feelings as well as realise I've got much better at handling this sort of situation than I used to be.

With some tics it's easy to see they're involuntary. With others it's harder, especially when they're triggered by the tensions friendships inevitably bring.

BRAIN MATTER

My recent ticcing fits haven't produced many funny moments so far. Today though, while I was writhing around having my sixth fit, an entire poem came out all in one go:

'My brain is made of flour,
My brain is made of dust,
My brain is made of cotton buds,
And horticultural fuss.'

Whether this is true or not remains to be seen. I'm not sure I could lie still enough for a brain scan at the moment.

THE BIG PUSH

PART ONE

A couple of weeks ago my appointment letter from wheelchair services arrived. My first reaction was one of sadness and fear. I wanted to cancel the appointment and throw the letter away, not because my mobility had improved, but because seeing it in black and white was upsetting. It felt like a step backwards. But within a few hours the feeling wore off, and now I feel much more positive about my appointment which is later today.

Walking about is very difficult because I drop to the ground a lot due to my leg tics. My movement is totally unpredictable and I need support from another person to get anywhere safely. Getting a wheelchair no longer feels like an option – it's become a necessity.

PART TWO

The woman who assessed me couldn't have been more lovely or thoughtful if she'd tried. She was amazingly in tune with the challenges my tics pose, both to walking around and when using a chair. She asked lots of questions about my life and measured me before bringing out a sample chair to try.

There are loads of different types of wheelchairs to choose from, and even when she'd decided which one was best for me she recommended lots of customisation to make sure it's able to withstand my wriggling.

I left feeling upbeat and hopeful. My chair will take about four weeks to prepare and adapt, then I can go back and see if it works. If everyone's happy that it does, I'll be allowed to take it home for road testing in my life.

FOOT BALLS

After a sudden flash of inspiration this evening I asked Leftwing Idiot to pass me a pen so I could write down my idea. Annoyingly, he didn't think I'd have enough control to take the pen from him safely, so he kept asking, 'Are you sure you're ready to take it, are you *sure?*'

With a long, irritated sigh I assured him I was.

He looked sceptical and handed the pen over slowly and cautiously. To his astonishment my hand grabbed the pen perfectly. As soon as it was in my hand though, my foot shot up and kicked him square in the balls.

He dropped to the floor with a heavy thud. I apologised repeatedly while he rolled around making strange noises that were a mixture of pain and laughter. Anyone would've thought he was having a fit.

MEANWHILE, BACK IN THE POST OFFICE

In front of me in the queue at the Post Office this morning was a boy of about eight with his mum. As usual I was ticcing a lot about biscuits and struggling to stand up. As the boy and his mum left he said 'Biscuit' under his breath. His mother whipped round and asked, 'Was that you?' He said it wasn't but she didn't believe him at all. 'That's not on,' she said and gave him a gentle clip round the ear.

I was pleased she hadn't ignored her son's behaviour, if a bit surprised by her approach. Perhaps Thump-A-Youth Man's teaching parenting skills in the area.

On my way out another young man was curious about all the biscuits. He was older and took a different approach. He asked Leftwing Idiot if I had Tourettes. 'Ask her,' he said, gesturing to me. I told him I had and he apologised, explaining that he'd never met anyone with Tourettes before. He was warm and friendly and I liked his open, straightforward attitude.

CHORES

I was at Leftwing Idiot's sitting on the sofa this afternoon while he was engrossed in something on his laptop. Without looking up he asked, 'What are you going to remind me to do later?' Absentmindedly I ticced some possible answers:

'Give Terry Waite a bath.'
'Take Michael Aspel out for a walk.'
'Take your washing out of the machine.'

I'll let you decide which was the correct answer.

GOODBYE, CARTOON STAR

The back room in Leftwing Idiot's flat, where I've been sleeping for the past few weeks, is the one with my favourite view in London. The big window looks out over several ramshackle gardens and the houses beyond. When I'm in bed all I can see is the vast sky, and I love going to sleep gazing up at it.

There's one star that's particularly bright, so bright it looks like the type of star a child would draw, with pointy rays stretching out into the darkness. My tics have named it 'cartoon star', and I frequently find myself talking to it while I'm going to sleep:

'Calm down, cartoon star.'
'Where are you cartoon star?'
'I love you cartoon star.'

I've been very happy staying with Leftwing Idiot. Today I've been thinking about some of the little things that have made me feel at home here, like cartoon star, the extra padding in the bathroom, all the strategically placed chairs, the amazing shared meals and morning songs – even the returned geranium!

In a week's time I'll be moving into my new lair with Poppy. It's exciting, and I'm looking forward to getting settled and finding out what my tics make of it all – I'm sure I'll be forging new relationships with inanimate objects, plants and burning suns from other galaxies.

'Goodnight cartoon star.'

LAYERS OF LOVELINESS

Last month I wrote about how my new ticcing fits had left me in a difficult situation. Lots of layers needed to be unpicked and sorted out to put me back in control. Now, nearly everything's been organised. I've got increased support from social services, full-time support at work, and a bright red emergency bag that goes everywhere with me. It feels like I'm getting back on track, even though the fits are still happening all the time.

My other big worry was how the fits would affect my move into the new lair. But now I have the right support in place they're not going to affect it at all, and in less than a week Poppy and I are moving in. I've spent the day with friends, making the new lair lovely. A lot of my stuff's there now – our new beds are ready, we have a shiny metal fridge, and I've got a new soft rug in the living room that's already been tic-tested.

I'm excited about moving in. It's taken a lot of organising, but something that felt impossible a month ago is happening now, thanks to help from my friends, and quick responses from the agencies that support me.

Layers of problems have been transformed into a safe and exciting move into the lovely new lair.

FIRST NIGHT AT THE CASTLE

Tonight's the first night in my new lair – affectionately known as the castle because it used to be a pub with that name. I love it and I've had a brilliant first evening here. Leftwing Idiot, King Russell and Bunny all came round. We had a delicious dinner and watched a film. Bunny's staying to provide my overnight care, so when I have a ticcing fit she'll be on hand to help.

When I first stepped inside the castle, before I bought it, I knew it was perfect, but I didn't think it would ever be possible for me to get to the stage where I could move in. But Leftwing Idiot told me you have to believe something's possible first and then look for ways to make it happen, otherwise you don't even bother trying. He was right and because I did what he suggested, I have a beautiful, accessible new home.

DECEMBER

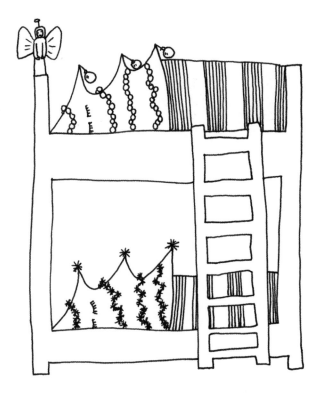

GOODNIGHT CHRISTMAS TREES

CREATIVITY CREEPS UP AT NIGHT

Sometimes my verbal ticcing fits don't produce much in the way of funny or interesting things, but the early hours of this morning provided a notable exception.

Bunny was providing my overnight care and I woke her just before 4am with a ticcing fit that went on for over an hour and a half. She successfully juggled making sure I was safe with frantically scribbling down the unexpected torrent of tics. I might not have been able to tell her how I was doing, but the words came flying out and kept us both laughing as dawn approached. She may have missed a few along the way, but Bunny filled three full pages of A4 with unexpected gems. Here's a selection:

'I overslept once, 44,000 million years ago.'

'The history of iguanas can be written in a teapot.'

'Hello darkness, my old bin.'

'What have you contributed to this conversation, mattress? You're more useless than a geranium.'

'Quiet, body: bears are trying to think in the woods.'

'Who's going to bother saving bins when we've got whales and energy to save?'

'I'm no friend of a leopard. I'm friend of a lion. I'm boasting about being friends with a lion.'

'Shadow puppet pissing in my hand.'

'Laser-beam me up, baby.'

'The clouds are chasing Helen Mirren.'

'The tree is feeling up the sky.'

'What's the difference between the air and a Basset hound? Twenty-six acres of wind.'

'I wonder if an owl got lost tonight.'

And Bunny's personal favourite: 'Bunny is the boss of bodies.'

It all ended just before 5:30am, after a lot of medication. Just as Bunny was leaving the room I ticced, 'If you see a barn owl, tell it to go away.'

When I look back at all these tics, I don't remember the discomfort of the fit, I'm just pleased that every so often amazing ideas emerge from such an uncomfortable experience.

COUNTS, SHOOTS AND LEAVES

I was sitting in Leftwing Idiot's kitchen this afternoon while he made some lunch for us both. While I waited for a sandwich I found myself absentmindedly counting the leaves on his geranium. It's not unusual for me to start counting stuff like this when I have a spare moment.

I hadn't planned on sharing this information with him because it's a habit I prefer to keep to myself. But while we were eating, I suddenly ticced, 'The geranium has 55 leaves.'

Leftwing Idiot laughed, looked across at me, and then the geranium, and said, 'That's true, isn't it?'

And of course it was.

LAMP POST IS THE NEW GERANIUM

Last summer my tics took against Leftwing Idiot's geranium for no apparent reason. Now I've moved into the castle they've found a new target – one that only comes out when it gets dark. My bedtime routine goes something like this: brush my teeth, get into bed, start verbally abusing the lamp post I can see from my window.

'Lamp post, stop glowing ostentatiously.'
'Lamp post, why are you loitering?'
'Lamp post, the trees laugh at you because you're short.'

I can't explain why this harmless piece of street furniture has become the focus of such venom. It may be because I don't have any blinds up yet and the light comes straight into my room.

This morning Poppy asked if I'll still abuse the lamp post when I've got some blinds. Leftwing Idiot laughed and said yes, I would. He then gave what I suspect is a fairly accurate prediction of what I might say:

'Lamp post, I know you're still out there.'
'Lamp post, why are you hiding?'

NOT DRUNK, DISORDERLY

Unusually, I'd not met the minicab driver who came to take me home before. When he saw me lurching towards the car he said to Bunny, who was helping me walk, 'No, no, no. Is she intoxicated?' I said I wasn't but he asked again, 'Are you drunk?' I said, 'No, I have Tourettes.'

He apologised instantly and profusely and continued to do so all the way home. He was still saying sorry when I had a ticcing fit in the back seat, but between apologies he was very thoughtful, asking Bunny if there was anything he could do to help.

He went on to tell us about his own experience of fits. His started when a motorbike accident he'd had in the '80s caused a serious brain injury. It meant he'd had multiple seizures every day for a very long time. But then, after ten years, they'd suddenly stopped and investigations revealed the damage had healed on its own.

It was an unexpectedly frank and personal account to be hearing from a stranger, and it made me wonder if my own ticcing fits might suddenly disappear one day.

AT HOME IN THE CASTLE

Christmas has come early at the castle. A couple of weeks ago an occupational therapist came to do an assessment of my needs. She made several recommendations, and today I've received a load of new equipment which should make life at home much easier and much safer.

I'm now the proud owner of a big blue inflatable bath seat. Its cushion inflates right up to the edge so I can slide onto it and then deflate it to lower myself into the water. When I've finished washing I can rise up again at the touch of a button so I no longer have to throw myself haphazardly out of the bath. Simple and brilliant!

Other new items include a fantastic wooden handrail which runs along the length of the hall. This makes moving from room to room easier and more elegant and, when no one's looking, I like to pretend I'm warming up in a ballet studio. My bed now has extra padding round the side to make thrashing about in the middle of the night that much less painful.

I've also added some stylish safety features of my own: a load of new cushions that offer perfect protection when I'm having a ticcing fit. Appropriately, these are all designed to look like biscuits.

A month ago I felt desperately sad and worried about the future. Now I feel at home and settled in my super, accessible, stylish castle.

CRUMBS

My least biscuity day in over a year is drawing to a close. After being a very regular part of my life for almost eighteen months my 'biscuit' tic suddenly seems to have stopped.

But I've had false alarms before about the end of the 'biscuit' era so it may still make a comeback. In the meantime, some other old favourites have stepped in to fill the crumbly void – it's been an especially big day for sheep-related tics:

'Fuck a sheep and eat its mother.'
'Don't fuck up the cheap sheep.'
'Fuck up a sheep and dance.'

SHOE CURE?

Poppy's mum is staying with us at the castle for a few days and this afternoon we went with Leftwing Idiot and some other friends to a local pub to check out their Christmas fair. On the way there I had a ticcing fit in a busy street.

It says a lot about how friendly the area is that, in the ten minutes the fit lasted, six or seven people stopped to ask if I was OK. Most of them were reassured by Leftwing Idiot's response, but one woman wasn't so easily satisfied. She insisted she knew how to help and repeatedly told him to take one of my shoes off and make me smell it. A bit of internet research revealed that this has long been an accepted treatment for epileptic seizures in some countries.

I'm happy to say Leftwing Idiot didn't follow her advice, although he did say he was thinking about trying it in future.

PECKHAM INSPIRES POETS

I went to the Post Office in Peckham with Bunny today. As we trudged back through the rain, my tics lifted our spirits with some rousing spontaneous versions of William Blake's famous poem 'Jerusalem'. Although we both enjoyed it to start with, two hours later when we were home and dry it was still coming out. By that time, I was exhausted and couldn't wait for it to stop.

Leftwing Idiot assures me William Blake saw angels in the trees on Peckham Rye. Clearly the Post Office nearby is my source of inspiration:

'And did those sheep in ancient times,
Talk about England's weathered past?
And did those sheep in ancient times, fuck up the sky?
No that was you, no that was you, no that was you, and I.
And in these deep and damaged times,
Who spilt courage on the floor?
And was a kitten killed here by dark satanic Heather Mills?
Bring me my sheep, Lizard man called Fred;
Bring me my Speedos of desire;
Bring me my chariot of Bill Gates' bum!
And what's left to do when all the dogs have died?
Fuck a sheep.'

ANGELS IN STOCKWELL

I went into town with Poppy this evening to do some Christmas shopping. I've hardly been using public transport at all recently because my ticcing fits are difficult to manage in busy places. However, the cost of cabs has been mounting, and as we were near Stockwell station we decided to travel by tube.

Just as we got through the ticket barrier I started to fit.

I've had some shoddy treatment on the underground in the past, in particular at Old Street station, but the staff at Stockwell couldn't have been more supportive and understanding. They took us behind the scenes to a safer, more private space and offered to help. But when Poppy told them we were fine and that we had an emergency plan, they let her get on with caring for me without making a fuss.

There are a couple of things that might help explain why I got a positive reaction from the Stockwell station staff (other than that they were just better informed). The first is that Poppy was with me and could explain what was happening, without ticcing. The second was that I was horizontal and clearly in need of help.

Since the ticcing fits started I've noticed how much friendlier and more concerned people are when I'm on the floor having a bad time, than they are when I'm vertical and asking for help.

Leftwing Idiot suggested we should create a Guide to Friendliness based on how many offers of assistance we get when I have a ticcing fit in different parts of town.

UN-KNOWLEDGE

I've mentioned a couple of times how I'm not very good at keeping secrets, and how this often means I tell people what gifts I've got them long before it's time to give them.

This problem got even worse today when Poppy told me what she's got Leftwing Idiot for Christmas. This is a massive responsibility and I'm doing my best to forget what she told me. But it's tricky to un-know something once you've been told.

THE TOURETTESMOBILE

This afternoon Leftwing Idiot and I went and picked up my new wheels. I'd had a call from the wheelchair clinic a couple of days ago to say my chair was ready and that I should come for a final fitting.

The appointment was with Maria, who'd carried out my original assessment, and William, a charismatic and enthusiastic technician. He was brilliant – he'd customised the chair so it meets my needs perfectly. He talked us through its features with a sales patter worthy of the best car showrooms. But because we have a national health service, this form of transport is mine free of charge.

William showed us all the extras he'd added for me, including a taller backrest, padded arms, and a four point seatbelt. The quick-release wheels were a particularly impressive surprise.

After William had taken the chair to pieces bit by bit, he turned to Leftwing Idiot and said, 'Now you put it back together!' Leftwing Idiot managed to do it, with William offering pointers and encouragement along the way.

All my previous worries that this would be an upsetting occasion proved unfounded, and it was exciting to sit in my new wheelchair for the first time. Thanks to Maria and William's kindness, energy and care, taking charge of the chair was an extremely positive experience. It'll give me greater freedom to make longer journeys and reduce the risk of injury both to me and to those who care for me.

Leftwing Idiot and I got the bus home – something we haven't been able to do at all easily for ages. With me securely in the chair everything felt much safer.

HOME ALONE

There was a gap this morning between my night support worker leaving and my Access to Work support worker – Bunny – arriving. This meant, for the first time since October when my ticcing fits started happening every day, I was on my own.

Leftwing Idiot lives very close by and he knew there was no one with me. I'd agreed with him that I'd stay on my bed until Bunny arrived and that if I got into trouble I'd phone him. Much as I love my friends and support workers, it felt exciting to be by myself for a bit.

But shortly before Bunny arrived a fit started. I managed to press the call button on my phone, which I'd kept on Leftwing Idiot's number. He answered immediately and could hear from the noise I was making that I was having a bad time. He hung up and was with me in less than two minutes.

Rather than being a failure, this feels like a success. It's showed that I can be by myself and call for help when I need it.

MARMOSET MOVES IN

A while ago I said that my long-standing biscuit tic was becoming increasingly rare, and although it hasn't gone completely, I'm saying it a lot less than I did. Instead I've been ticcing a lot about sheep, women, and a strange Tourettes invention: the 'Win-Bin'.

Over the last few days another word has crept in: 'marmoset'. I'd no idea what a marmoset was, but with the help of the internet I was able to establish that my new visitor's a species of monkey.

Bunny was supporting me at work today and she particularly enjoyed this cheeky new tic. While we ate lunch she said wistfully, 'I wish I could just say "marmoset" all the time without sounding fake.' I really loved that she felt this way and my tics threw in a few more monkeys as a reward.

Lots of people say they wish they had Tourettes so they could shout swear words in public. This is thoughtless and I've never heard any of my friends say anything like it. But many people who know me do have favourite tics. Leftwing Idiot told me he often says my tics out loud when I'm not around because he enjoys how they sound, and saying them cheers him up.

How long my troop of monkey tics will hang around for before swinging back to the jungle is anyone's guess – my tics are delightfully unpredictable.

SPIRITED AWAY

Poppy and I went to the shops today, with me in my wheelchair. I kept ticcing at the top of my voice, 'I'm being punished for being a sinner!' and 'I have an evil spirit inside me!'

I've no idea why these tics suddenly surfaced, but I do know from previous experience that this is exactly what some people think is happening when they see and hear me. On the occasions when strangers have told me I'm possessed and in need of exorcism, I've generally found it upsetting (if sometimes amusing) and difficult to respond to. Hearing my own tics play up to this idea made Poppy and me laugh.

It reminded me of a time Leftwing Idiot had told me about when he was with a friend who has cerebral palsy and uses a wheelchair. They saw a couple on the street looking nervous at their approach. Leftwing Idiot whispered to his friend, 'Go on, do your disabled impression.' She took great pleasure in doing this, making a loud noise, jerking her arms around, and generally playing up to the stereotypical image of a disabled person in a wheelchair. The couple jumped with shock and hurried past, much to the amusement of Leftwing Idiot and his friend.

Sometimes, playing with negative preconceptions of disability can be fun, and having a laugh about it with friends can help neutralise the impact of bad interactions.

THE UNSPOKEN TRUTH

Accessible toilets always stink of shit.

I'll let that sink in for a moment.

In the meantime, you might have noticed I'm referring to accessible toilets rather than disabled toilets. This isn't just me being super PC, it's a question of accuracy – a toilet can only really be disabled if the flush is missing or something.

Anyway, it doesn't seem to matter where the accessible toilet is or how well it's looked after, it almost always has the lingering smell of poo. This is probably because many non-disabled people think accessible toilets are a good place to have a sneaky dump as they're more private and less frequently used than ordinary conveniences. I've got no proof of this of course, but I do have extensive experience of accessible toilets. And it's not always because I need the loo. Sometimes, when I'm having a tic-cing fit, accessible toilets provide a very welcome refuge for me. But whatever the reason, I've spent a lot more time rolling about on the floors of accessible toilets than is ideal lately.

Rigorous research has been carried out into accessible toilets by a team at University College London. They produced 'The Accessible Toilet Resource', which explains why accessible public toilets are important and provides detailed advice on good prac-tice for design. Their audit of accessible toilets doesn't mention smell but does identify other common problems including clut-ter, cleanliness and poorly fitted grab rails.

So next time you find yourself sloping off to the accessible toilet for a surreptitious dump, spare a thought for the disabled person who's waiting to use it after you.

'NICE UP YOUR CHRISTMAS TREE'

Last night Poppy and I decorated the Christmas tree in the castle and this afternoon I went to our end of year parties at work – first for the kids and then for the staff.

As we edge closer and closer to Christmas and the end of the year, I can't help but reflect on the changes, challenges, and opportunities the last twelve months have brought.

At the kids' party this afternoon I sat by the bonfire, sending excited children off on a festive treasure hunt. That was a real privilege, made possible only because of my support worker and the emergency bag by my side.

Earlier on I'd got frustrated when I tried to unlock a door and my hand wouldn't co-operate because of my tics. For a moment I let the frustration overwhelm me and I hit the door with my fist. This is the sort of regular annoyance my tics provoke, but over-reacting in the way I did happens a lot less than it used to. That's because, although some things have got worse for me (like having problems walking and the ticcing fits), other aspects have got better. I'm certainly getting more help than I was this time last year, and I'm more confident about asking for it when I need it. I'm sleeping better, eating better and generally being more honest about the things I find hard.

I still have a few days of work left before I stop for the year, but I'm really looking forward to my first Christmas in the castle – which is looking very festive, thanks to Poppy's enthusiastic work on the tree.

A STAMPEDE

My tics often drift onto the topic of celebrities such as Ronan Keating, making wild unfounded accusations such as 'In the Night Garden Ronan Keating flashed his underwear.' Or, more ominously, suggesting 'I'd like Ronan Keating's heart on a stake.' In reality I've got nothing against singers like Ronan, and this afternoon I got a glimpse of what life in a boy band would be like for myself.

It happened on my way to lunch with Bunny when I dropped to the ground with a ticcing fit in a back alley near my office. I've often had fits in public and there are often passers-by who ask if I'm OK, but also lots who don't.

The alley wasn't a great place to be fitting – the ground was hard and covered in glass. It did, however, turn out to be the friendliest place in London, with loads of different people offering their assistance one after the other. Bunny calmly explained that the fits happened several times a day and that we were fine and had everything we needed.

While I was on the floor having a rough time I saw a group of ten or so young women from the local college running towards me. For a moment I wondered where they were going before realising I was their destination, and that they were rushing to help me. Anyone who says London is an unfriendly place clearly hasn't rolled around in an alley in Stockwell.

WAITING ROOM HEARTS AND MINDS

One of the last-minute things Leftwing Idiot and I had to do before Christmas was go to the chemist to pick up a prescription so I have enough medication to see me through the holidays.

The surgery normally send my prescription direct to the pharmacist to make things easier, but this time there'd been some miscommunication between the two which meant I had to wait in the chemist's much longer than I'd expected.

The chemist was very busy and I wasn't the only person waiting. Though it's only a small shop, there's a huddled row of four chairs for people waiting to get their prescriptions. I sat on one, and three women sat quietly in the others.

I could sense the women were unnerved by my tics and didn't know what to make of me. After about ten minutes one of them beckoned to Leftwing Idiot. She asked him in a hushed voice, but still completely audible to me, 'Is she in pain when she makes that noise?' Leftwing Idiot said she could ask me. I smiled and explained the tics were mostly just uncomfortable. Like when I explain to children, I compared it to the sensation of trying to hold back a sneeze.

The atmosphere in the crowded shop eased immediately. The women, who'd seemed to be scowling before, were now all smiles. It was a perfect reminder of how easily and quickly attitudes can change for the better and how often this starts with someone being curious enough to ask a question.

As we left, everyone cheerfully wished us a happy Christmas.

TOUCHED BY THE PAST

At this time of year people's thoughts tend to drift back to their childhoods, and I was prompted to think about mine yesterday by a ticcing fit.

Last night, just as a long fit was drawing to a close, I noticed one of my fingers waggling ferociously backwards and forwards. Given how much wriggling the rest of my body does this shouldn't have been surprising, but seeing and feeling it reminded me it was something that used to happen in exactly the same way when I was about eleven.

I had fewer, less noticeable tics when I was a kid, but I remember finding this finger-waggling particularly odd, mainly because it felt so automatic and unstoppable. I even remember telling a physiotherapist who was treating an injury to my arm about it, but she wasn't interested. After a few months it stopped and I've not thought about it since – at least not until last night, when my finger started waggling again.

This wasn't the only strange recollection invoked by the fit. Another was about my feet. They'd tensed up, which led Leftwing Idiot to try tickling them. He was surprised by my lack of response, even during a fit, and asked me if I could feel the various parts of my feet he was prodding. Although I knew he was touching the soles, the sensation wasn't very specific and I couldn't tell exactly where his finger was.

This too was very familiar. I told him my family have long believed I have poor sensitivity in my hands and feet. This was noticed first when I was about seven by a physio who was assessing me because my first primary school was concerned about my co-ordination and how I moved. She suggested my parents rub my hands and feet with an electric toothbrush, which my dad dutifully did for years.

I've never been convinced about this lack of sensitivity, mainly because I've never known any different. On holidays, though, I'd always get back to the beach with the soles of my feet cut to shreds because I'd not noticed how sharp the rocks were.

My mum didn't like the idea of me being medically labelled but she was concerned enough to take me to see a neurologist. He told her I was just a clumsy, unco-ordinated child. I was already very aware that I moved and behaved differently from my school friends, and I even started the 'Clumsy Cleo Club', named after a character in a story tape I loved, to help me fit in.

But it wasn't as simple as just being clumsy. I was chaotic and hard to teach and had a diagnosis of dyslexia and dyspraxia. My first school struggled with my behaviour and when I was eight they said they couldn't meet my needs. They told my parents if I stayed, they wouldn't move me up to the next class with my peers.

My mum took the decision to move me to a different school. The new one specialised in teaching children with learning and behavioural difficulties, supporting them back into mainstream education. They gave me specialist input and support, and carefully rebuilt my confidence. I was only there for two years, but the school transformed me.

Tourettes wasn't known about much when I was a child, and with hindsight it's clear some of the things I did or said back then were tics. But my parents were very accepting of my unusual behaviour and didn't want it medicalised. I once asked my dad why I did certain things or found particular things hard, and he explained that I was just 'wired differently'.

Although I'd shown him some of my school reports, I'd not talked in detail to Leftwing Idiot about any of this until last night when my memory was jogged by a waggling finger and a scrunched-up foot.

FESTIVE GERANIUMS

Today's a very special day because it's the only day of the year my regular 'Happy Christmas' tic is appropriate and in context – so, Happy Christmas!

Fat Sister's gift from the NHS (her employer) is three fourteen-hour shifts – including one today. Despite this she's in good spirits. She and King Russell stayed at the castle last night, and they'll be here for the next few days as well.

While Fat Sister's at work King Russell and I will be hanging out, watching films and eating. We've already opened some presents this morning but we'll wait until Fat Sister gets home to do the rest.

Leftwing Idiot's off having lunch with his parents. He called this morning to wish me a Happy Christmas but ended up goading me with joyful descriptions of how festive his geranium's looking – he'd decorated it with a ribbon round its pot, and some tinsel. It was difficult to claim I'm really not bothered by this plant when my tics were interrupting with advice like, 'Tangle its roots with tinsel.'

For a lot of people Christmas is a time for family, friends, food, and thoughtfulness. My first Christmas at the castle's been full of all these things, as well as some unwelcome geranium-based conversation.

Because now's the only time my festive tics can run free without sounding strange, I'm going to end with a selection of my favourites:

'Happy Christmas my biscuits.'
'Mind control to Major Christmas.'
'Happy Christmas dear otter.'
'I'd like to see Christmas trees docking themselves on the moon.'
'Goodnight Christmas trees.'

ON THE EVE OF AN ENDING

This time last year I made a resolution – to look for ways to acknowledge and celebrate my tics, rather than ignore them and the increasing impact they were having on my life. I'm proud to say I've stuck with it through thick and thin, and it's been better for me than any New Year's resolution I've ever made.

During the last twelve months there have been some seriously tricky times, as well as many high points. A year ago I was more mobile and I wasn't having the explosive ticcing fits that have come to dominate the last few months. But my face and chest were constantly bruised from my relentless motor tics, and I didn't have the confidence to talk about Tourettes without tears.

During the last six weeks I've spent over 113 hours having ticcing fits – an average of almost three hours a day. That's obviously a lot, but when I looked at a recent survey that shows how people in this country use their time, I discovered it's less than the time the average person spends sitting on the sofa.

Perhaps more shockingly, most people spend an average of only 6 minutes a day laughing. Thanks to Tourettes, I know my friends and I laugh a lot more than this. Hopefully, reading this book will have bumped up your average too.

Today, some people will see my wheelchair, my support worker and my fits as signs that things have got worse. The thing is, they don't *feel* worse. There have been plenty of tough times lately, but with the help of friends, professionals and even strangers, I feel amazingly well supported and ready for whatever challenges and opportunities the next twelve months may bring.

A year on, I'm taking this opportunity to reflect on some key moments in my transformation from Tourettes *sufferer* into Tourettes*hero*.

DECIDING TO BE DIFFERENT

Exactly 364 days ago I chose to record my tics for twenty-four hours and share my experiences of living with Tourettes in writing. I didn't realise at the time what a significant turning point this would be. Ignoring my tics wasn't working, and my confidence was slipping as I struggled to cope. My resolution last New Year's Eve was to tackle Tourettes head on and make it my power, not my problem.

CELEBRATING STRANGERS

In February I met Thump-A-Youth Man and he recounted an incident in which (without me knowing) he'd thumped someone who'd been laughing at me on a bus. Hearing this made me realise how many unusual and surreal discussions I'd had, prompted by Tourettes. It helped me rethink my interactions with strangers and realise they give me opportunities for amazing conversations – something most people don't get the chance to have.

PRACTICAL SOLUTIONS

Discovering Access to Work and choosing the perfect pair of padded gloves were just two of the practical solutions that helped shift my approach to Tourettes. Rather than trying to 'fix things' by using drugs, I started to focus on simple solutions to limit the impact of tics on my life. I've realised most problems are solvable if you get creative, and I feel more confident and in control as a result.

TAKING TOUGH DECISIONS

When faced with a difficult situation it's all too easy to ignore it and put off addressing it. My instinct had been to ignore my dete-riorating mobility, but thankfully my friends wouldn't allow this to happen. My decision to move from the lair to the castle felt incredibly daunting at the time, but I can't imagine how much harder things would have been if I'd stayed put. The castle's given me the accessibility I need to maintain my freedom with-out risk. I sat in the kitchen early this evening and felt overcome with love for my new home.

Although there have been major changes, moves and marriages during the year, some things have stayed the same.

There's the shared laughter with Laura, the joy of hanging out with Poppy, the unstinting loyalty and love of Fat Sister, the con-sistent care of King Russell, and my enduring friendship with Leftwing Idiot – whose ongoing support has made my life with Tourettes easier and happier.

And of course there have been the tics – rude, funny, shocking, poetic, biscuity and surreal, but always a surprise. It seems right to let them have the last word:

'The bashing branches of a boring sycamore on a night in December give way to a fairytale universe in January.'

Happy New Year!

Visit www.touretteshero.com to continue the journey.

FREQUENTLY ASKED QUESTIONS

WHAT IS TOURETTES?

Gilles de la Tourette Syndrome (Tourettes) is a neurological condition. It's estimated to affect more than 300,000 children and adults in the UK, and I'm one of them. 'Tics' are a key feature of Tourettes – these are the involuntary and uncontrollable sounds and movements people with Tourettes make. The sounds are called vocal tics and the movements are called motor tics. Tourettes is three times more common in males than it is in females, so I'm three times more unusual than most.

WHAT CAUSES TOURETTES?

The cause of Tourettes isn't known, but current research suggests it involves a part of the brain called the basal ganglia and a dysfunction of the neurotransmitters (chemical messengers in the brain). There's also strong evidence to suggest it's an inherited condition. At least one other person in my close family has tics too.

WHY DO PEOPLE WITH TOURETTES SWEAR?

Most people with Tourettes don't swear. This aspect of Tourettes only affects 10% of people who have it. But there's coprolalia and copropraxia, and I have both. Coprolalia means using obscene or unacceptable language. Copropraxia means making obscene or otherwise unacceptable movements or gestures. Sometimes I end up doing both at once.

ARE YOU POSSESSED?

Believe it or not, I'm asked this fairly regularly. Some people think the movements and noises of my tics indicate I'm possessed by a demon. But the simple answer is no, I'm not. I usually respond to this question by asking why an evil spirit would make me go around shouting about biscuits.

HOW IS TOURETTES DIAGNOSED?

For Tourettes to be diagnosed, multiple motor tics and at least one vocal tic must be present over a period of a year without a break of more than three months. I tic thousands of times a day and they're very noticeable. Observing and evaluating symptoms is the only way to diagnose Tourettes, but there are rating scales to help assess the severity of people's tics.

WHAT TREATMENTS ARE AVAILABLE?

While there's no cure, there are some treatments available that can help control the symptoms. There's a wide range of drugs, which includes anti-psychotics, anti-hyperactives and anti-depressants, but none that has been developed specifically for Tourettes.

Individuals react differently to different drugs, and while these may be successful for some people, they don't work for everybody, and can have undesirable side effects.

Other types of treatment include behavioural therapies like Habit Reversal Therapy (HRT) and Comprehensive Behavioural Intervention Therapy (CBIT). These aim to improve people's awareness of their tics and teach alternative movements that have less impact. Research from the US published in 2010 showed that behavioural treatments can be as effective as drugs in managing the symptoms of Tourettes.

Deep brain stimulation is a neurosurgical procedure that places a stimulator in the brain. It's used to treat other movement disorders such as Parkinson's and is currently being trialled in the UK for Tourettes.

IS TOURETTES ASSOCIATED WITH ANY OTHER CONDITIONS?

Over 85% of people with Tourettes have more than just tics. Common additional conditions (known as co-morbidities) include: Attention Deficit Hyperactivity Disorder (ADHD) and Obsessive Compulsive Disorder (OCD).

For some people, co-morbidities may present more problems than the tics themselves even if they're less visible.

I don't have a diagnosis of OCD but I do have some obsessive and compulsive behaviour.

WHAT ARE TICS?

Tics are chronic (long-term) repetitive and involuntary sounds and movements. It's possible to suppress tics for a while, but eventually they have to be let out. Tics usually start in childhood around the age of seven.

For some people, symptoms disappear as they get older, but for many, Tourettes carries on into adulthood. Tics can be as simple as blinking, grimacing or coughing, or as complex as jumping, or uttering complete phrases. Tics can be experienced in lots of different ways by the same person. They can change over time and get more or less intense in different situations.

Some people find their tics reduce during absorbing activities. I sometimes tic less when I'm concentrating on drawing (like the ones in this book) or when I'm swimming. Changes in tic severity and frequency are unpredictable, and this is part of the challenge of living with Tourettes.

WHAT DO TICS FEEL LIKE?

People with Tourettes describe what their tics feel like in different ways. For me, different tics have different sensations. Some feel like I'm being yanked from the inside, others are more like a pressure building up that needs to be released – like a sneeze.

Both feel as though they're happening in specific parts of my body. The worst tics affect the whole of my body and feel like all of my insides are itching and can't be scratched.

WHAT'S A MOTOR TIC?

Motor tics are involuntary movements. These can include blinking, shrugging, jumping, twirling, head jerking, leg bending, eye rolling, and grimacing.

Sometimes motor tics can make everyday activities like eating or typing extremely difficult. My leg tics have made walking so difficult I often use a wheelchair to get around.

WHAT'S A VOCAL (OR PHONIC) TIC?

Vocal tics are involuntary noises or words. These can include whistling, squeaking, sniffing, coughing, yelping, screaming, uttering words or phrases – and for some people, swearing.

When I'm talking to people my vocal tics can interrupt so much it's hard to express myself clearly. Sometimes, though, vocal tics are extremely funny – and that's when things start to get interesting.

WHY DO CERTAIN WORDS BECOME TICS?

It's a mystery. Tics vary greatly from person to person, but any movement, word or sound can become a tic.

ARE VOCAL TICS SAYING WHAT YOU'RE THINKING?

No. To describe Tourettes as a condition that makes you say what you're thinking would be oversimplifying it. Most tics are totally random. This doesn't mean they're never triggered by what's going on around you, because sometimes they are.

Tics tend not to be related to the actual thoughts or feelings of the person who has them. Tics can sometimes involve saying the most inappropriate thing in a situation: for example, making a comment about someone's appearance or giving away a secret. I sometimes catch myself shouting out my pin number when I'm using a cash machine (but don't tell anyone).

DO TICS HURT?

This is a difficult question to answer. The sensations that trigger tics can be very uncomfortable – particularly if I try and hold them in. And the consequences of ticcing can be painful too, like when I bang my chest or head-butt a table. The same tic can hurt more or less depending on where I am. For example, dropping to my knees on a carpet hurts a lot less than on concrete.

WHAT'S A TICCING FIT?

I use the term ticcing fit to describe a distinct period of over-powering and constant motor tics. Fits generally last between 10 minutes and an hour, although the longest was just over three hours and required emergency treatment in hospital. During these fits any part of my body may move, shake, contort or lock into painful positions.

My fits look a bit like an epileptic seizure, but there are some key differences. I stay fully conscious and know what's happening around me, and although I can't always speak I can usually communicate in some way with whoever's helping me.

Most of the time these fits can be managed with the help of a friend or support worker. I always carry an emergency bag containing my medical information, medication, and the protective clothing I need for when they occur. They can happen at any time of the day or night, and without someone being with me I'm very likely to injure myself.

I'm currently having about eight of these fits every day. Although they're exhausting and put a huge strain on my body, once they've stopped I'm immediately fine and can carry on with whatever I was doing before.

WHAT ARE ECHOPHENOMENA?

These specific types of tic involve echoing or repeating sounds, words or movements.

Echolalia means repeating other people's sounds or speech.

Echopraxia means repeating other people's gestures or movements.

Palilalia is similar to echolalia but involves someone repeating their own sounds or speech.

Rambolalia and *discolalia* are terms my tics made up for their own amusement and I'm not sure what they mean exactly.

WHAT DO YOU DO WHEN PEOPLE STARE, LAUGH OR MAKE COMMENTS?

People with Tourettes choose to deal with other people's reactions in different ways. Most people I meet are friendly and understanding about Tourettes. When people respond less positively and laugh, stare, or make negative comments, I challenge them and do my best to explain. This can often lead to a change in their attitude, and I've had many great conversations that have started this way.

There will always be some people who don't change their attitude, or who continue to be mean and sometimes aggressive. In these situations I ignore their behaviour and try not to get upset or angry myself.

DO YOU EVER SAY STUFF ON PURPOSE AND PRETEND YOU DIDN'T MEAN TO?

This is something people with Tourettes are often accused of. I can't speak for anyone else, but I've never claimed something was a tic when it wasn't. Tics tend to sound different from my normal speaking voice and most people who know me can tell the difference without needing to ask.

DOES HAVING TOURETTES AFFECT THE WAY YOU SLEEP?

Yes. Tourettes can have a big impact on how well somebody sleeps. Tics make it hard for me to stay still and quiet enough to get to sleep. Staying asleep can be difficult too. While most people don't tic in their sleep, mine often wake me up in the middle of the night so I use a weighted blanket to help me stay as still as possible.

HOW DO YOU MANAGE AT WORK?

People with Tourettes do all sorts of different jobs, and how they manage depends on their individual circumstances. I'm open and honest about my tics with my employer and colleagues and they give me a lot of support. I always explain that I have Tourettes to new people I meet at work and tell them it's fine to ask questions about it.

I also get help from Access to Work, which pays for the support that disabled people in employment may need to do their jobs. For me, this scheme pays for the majority of my travel costs to and from work, and for a personal assistant to help me while I'm there.

ARE THERE ANY THINGS YOU DON'T DO BECAUSE YOU HAVE TOURETTES?

Tourettes can easily become a socially isolating condition. It's important for me that I don't let it dictate the sort of activities I'm able to enjoy. I do this by making sure I plan carefully and have the right support when I do stuff. Having lots of close friends is important to me too.

Sometimes I change how I do practical things to make sure I stay safe, and there are only a few things I don't do at all, like using sharp knives or tools, or carrying breakable objects.

DO YOU PREFER PEOPLE TO IGNORE OR ACKNOWLEDGE YOUR TICS?

My personal preference is for people to respond openly to my tics. Tourettes isn't funny but lots of tics are. If I say something that's particularly surreal or shocking, I think it's right for people to acknowledge it.

Most of the time, though, I prefer my tics to be ignored. Lots of people tell me that once they've got used to them, they're able to tune them out altogether. If I need practical help because of a motor tic I'll ask for it, and I'm always happy when people offer to give me a hand.

WHAT SHOULD I DO IF I THINK I, OR SOMEONE I KNOW, MAY HAVE TOURETTES?

I've had tics since childhood, but it took me a long time to seek a medical opinion. My parents worried about people labelling me or discriminating against me, and were reluctant for me to be formally diagnosed. But I've never regretted seeking help with understanding something that's been a big part of my life for as long as I can remember. The diagnosis has meant that I'm able to access the support I need to manage my tics and reduce their impact.

My advice for anyone who thinks they or someone they know has Tourettes would be:

- Read up on Tourettes – a good place to start would be the Tourettes Action website, www.tourettes-action.org.uk
- If it's appropriate, discuss your thoughts and concerns with your friends and family.
- Speak to your GP and ask for a referral to a specialist neurologist. Be persistent and remember, your GP may not be as familiar with Tourettes as you are.
- It helps to keep a record of all vocal and motor tics. Some people find keeping a video diary is useful for this.

Living with Tourettes has many challenges, but with the right support, understanding and encouragement, these can usually be overcome.

While it can be difficult, having Tourettes has made me a more empathetic, resilient, confident and articulate person.

And remember, if you are diagnosed with Tourettes, you'll be in good company.